Praise

"Schiller does an amazing [...] cism and spirituality, science [...] of dreamwork/studies."
—**DEBORAH L. KORN, PSYD,** clinical psychologist, faculty member at Trauma Research Foundation and EMDR Institute, and coauthor of *Every Memory Deserves Respect*

"A rare combination of scholarship and fascinating insight about generational trauma gained from personal experience and therapeutic practice."
—**J. M. DEBORD,** author of *The Dream Interpretation Dictionary*

"Our dreams are one of the most potent ways to receive [our ancestors'] messages.…Linda Schiller's incredible book *Ancestral Dreaming* gives us the keys to unlock our most profound inheritance."
—**DR. KELLY SULLIVAN WALDEN,** author of *Dreamifesting* and host of *The Kelly Walden Show*

"A remarkable journey through ancestral whispers, dreams, wounds, and blessings."
—**DR. CLARE JOHNSON,** author of *Elixir of Sleep* and *The Art of Lucid Dreaming*

"Schiller masterfully guides seekers on the path of ancestral healing through dreams."
—**SHELLEY A. KAEHR, PHD,** author of *Ancestral Energy Healing*

"A fascinating journey through ancestral healing, dreamwork, and the deep connections that bind past, present, and future."
—**DEIRDRE BARRETT, PHD,** author of *The Committee of Sleep* and president of IASD

"Linda possesses a remarkable ability to clearly make sense of complex material.…This book will be an invaluable resource."
—**DAVID KAHN, PHD,** psychiatry instructor at Harvard Medical School and executive committee adviser to IASD

"As a fan of Linda's relaxed, friendly writing, her broad counseling approach, and deep mystic insights, I am blown away by her new book."
—**STASE MICHAELS,** author of *Nightmares*

"A comprehensive yet intimate approach."
—**BENJAMIN STIMPSON,** therapist and author of *Ancestral Whispers*

"Linda's latest book helps us sort out ancestral influences to see where they are holding us back and where they are sources of personal strength and resilience."
—**KATHERINE R. BELL, PHD,** host of *The Dream Journal* podcast

"Schiller provides exercises in support of those who want to begin to walk the path of an ancestrally informed dream-worker…with clarity and compassionate encouragement."
—**DR. KIMBERLY MASCARO,** author of *Dreaming with the Earth-Mind*

"Linda invokes a multi-cultural, multi-theoretical foundation with which to evoke our own mythic connections and longings."
—**JULIE LEAVITT, DMIN, BC-DMT, LMHC,** professor at Lesley University, Hebrew College, and Hebrew Union College

"Schiller demonstrates how, by recognizing intergenerational impact… readers can confront their fears and break harmful patterns."
—**VICTORIA RABINOWE,** director of DreamingArts Studio in Santa Fe and faculty on the JungPlatform

"A joy to read.…Schiller's thorough investigation into our connections to the departed builds a method for understanding our own motivations."
—**WALTER BERRY,** author of *Drawn into the Dream*

"Schiller offers a creative and practical approach to discovering our biological and spiritual ancestors.…This book offers an anchoring sense of presence and hope for deep healing."
—**TZIVIA GOVER,** certified dreamwork professional and author of *Dreaming on the Page*

"I was particularly excited to learn about Linda Schiller's spiritual approach to explore ancestors' dreams because she incorporates the wisdom of the body to explore further layers of meaning."
—MAG. JOHANNA VEDRAL, lecturer at Sigmund Freud University, psychologist, and author of *Collage Dream Writing*

"If you are interested in how your dreams connect you to your ancestral heritage, Linda Schiller offers a very thorough and practical book on how to do just that."
—DR. LESLIE ELLIS, author of *A Clinician's Guide to Dream Therapy*

"Schiller builds a clear and heartfelt bridge between dreaming and ancestral legacy."
—JORDI BORRAS, founder of Mondesomnis ("Dream World"), leader of the Dream Integration Program, and psychotherapist

"Schiller's deep dive into intergenerational healing through dream work isn't just an outstanding book. It's a calling."
—BETH RONTAL, LICSW, psychotherapist

"Practical, highly readable, and full of deep wisdom."
—RYAN HURD, author of *Lucid Talisman* and *Sleep Paralysis*

"Schiller offers a profound roadmap for this healing journey.... [She] is a brilliant guide to help us navigate toward light, integration, and peace."
—LAUREN Z. SCHNEIDER, MFT, author of *Tarotpy - It's All in the Cards*

Ancestral Dreaming

About the Author

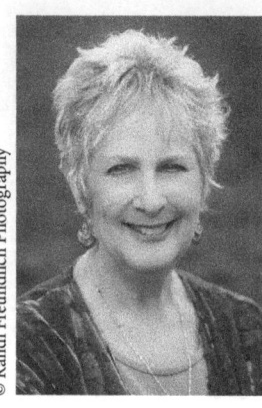
© Randi Freundlich Photography

Linda Yael Schiller, MSW, LICSW is an international speaker and author on dreamwork, trauma, and integrated embodied spiritually, an integrative mind/body/spiritual psychotherapist and consultant with over forty years' experience, and a long-term member of The International Association for the Study of Dreams. She is the author of *Ancestral Dreaming: Heal Generational Wounds Through Dreamwork* (2025), *PTSDreams: Transform Your Nightmares from Trauma through Healing Dreamwork* (2022), *Modern Dreamwork: New Tools for Decoding Your Soul's Wisdom* (2019), and *Comprehensive and Integrative Trauma Treatment Workbook* (Western Schools, 2010), as well as numerous articles and book chapters. Linda is also trained in the body/mind methodologies of EMDR, EFT, TAT, HBLU, Kabbalah healing, Enneagram, hypnotherapy, Somatic Experiencing, Focusing, and Reiki.

As Professor Emeritus at Boston University School of Social Work and Simmons University, she has received awards for her original theory of relational group work, and recognition worldwide for her teaching excellence.

Linda regularly teaches dreamwork and facilitates dream groups on her original dreamwork methods, which include her "Integrated Embodied Dreamwork" approach, her unique "Dreamwork through the Lens of Kabbalah," which includes the Pardes Method of layers of dream meaning, and her nightmare protocol based on best-practice trauma treatment and Jungian active imagination called "The GAIA Method: A Guided Active Imagination Approach."

She is a vibrant, warm, and dynamic speaker and has been described as "engaging, articulate, and inspiring." Linda has been a member of her own dream circle for over forty years.

www.lindayaelschiller.com
lindayschiller@gmail.com
https://www.facebook.com/linda.schiller.9461
https://www.instagram.com/lindayschiller22/

Ancestral Dreaming

Heal Generational Wounds Through Dreamwork

LINDA YAEL SCHILLER

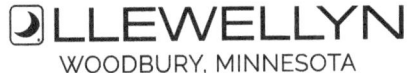
WOODBURY, MINNESOTA

Ancestral Dreaming: Heal Generational Wounds Through Dreamwork Copyright © 2025 by Linda Yael Schiller. All rights reserved. No part of this book may be used or reproduced in any manner whatsoever, including internet usage, without written permission from Llewellyn Worldwide Ltd., except in the case of brief quotations embodied in critical articles and reviews. No part of this book may be used or reproduced in any manner for the purpose of training artificial intelligence technologies or systems.

First Edition
First Printing, 2025

Book design by Samantha Peterson
Cover design by Shannon McKuhen
Interior illustrations by Llewellyn Art Department
Vagus nerve illustration on page 122: The brain, in right profile with the glossopharyngeal and vagus nerves and, to the right, a view of the base of the brain. Photolithograph from 1940 after a 1543 woodcut. Wellcome Collection. Public Domain Mark (page 3)

Llewellyn Publications is a registered trademark of Llewellyn Worldwide Ltd.

Library of Congress Cataloging-in-Publication Data (Pending)
ISBN: 978-0-7387-7891-4

Llewellyn Worldwide Ltd. does not participate in, endorse, or have any authority or responsibility concerning private business transactions between our authors and the public.

All mail addressed to the author is forwarded but the publisher cannot, unless specifically instructed by the author, give out an address or phone number.

Any internet references contained in this work are current at publication time, but the publisher cannot guarantee that a specific location will continue to be maintained. Please refer to the publisher's website for links to authors' websites and other sources.

Note: The information in this book is not meant to diagnose, treat, prescribe, or substitute consultation with a licensed mental health professional.

Llewellyn Publications
A Division of Llewellyn Worldwide Ltd.
2143 Wooddale Drive
Woodbury, MN 55125-2989
www.llewellyn.com

Printed in the United States of America

GPSR Representation:
UPI-2M PLUS d.o.o., Medulićeva 20, 10000 Zagreb, Croatia,
matt.parsons@upi2mbooks.hr

Other Books by Linda Yael Schiller

Comprehensive and Integrative Trauma Treatment Workbook

Modern Dreamwork
New Tools for Decoding Your Soul's Wisdom

PTSDreams
*Transform Your Nightmares from
Trauma through Healing Dreamwork*

To my family and dear friends,
especially Steve and Sara.

Contents

List of Exercises ... xiii

Introduction ... 1

Chapter 1: What Are Your Ancestors Telling You or Asking of You? ... 13

Chapter 2: Bring Home My Bones ... 39

Chapter 3: Epigenetics and Healing the Dreams We Carry from Others ... 49

Chapter 4: Respecting Dreamwork and Ancestry Worldwide, and the Unique Work of Ancestry with Adoption ... 67

Chapter 5: Griefwork and Ancestors ... 85

Chapter 6: The Embodied Nature of Trauma, Nightmares, and Intergenerational Trauma Transmission ... 105

Chapter 7: GAIA Method Applied to Ancestral Dreams and Nightmares ... 133

Chapter 8: Your Ancestral Tasks: Honoring, Healing, Returning, Remembering ... 161

Chapter 9: Conversations, Compassion, and Creativity for Ancestral Healing ... 187

Chapter 10: How to Become a Wise and Good Future Ancestor ... 201

Acknowledgments ... 209

Bibliography ... 213

Exercises

Building Your Genogram ... 10
Creating a Sapphire-Blue Container of Light ... 17
Identifying Old Grudges ... 31
Dream Incubation to Connect with Ancestors ... 34
Bone-Knowing ... 46
Catching the Repeats ... 53
Letting Go of the Rocks ... 62
Gratitude Practice ... 64
Helping Tangled Spirits Over the Threshold ... 91
Recognizing and Discerning Your Ancestors ... 102
Sapphire Light Boundaries and Your Posse of Protection ... 108
Grounding in the Present and Attaching ... 112
"I Feel, I Am" ... 125
Shaking It Off ... 127
Safe Place Imagery ... 143
Gathering Your Posse ... 144
Sunray Association Circle ... 148
Using the GAIA Method ... 156
Reaching Out Through All the Realms ... 164
Find Your Wise and Well Elder ... 174
Protection When Working with Angry Ancestors ... 179
Boundary Balancing Technique ... 182
Sending Them Back ... 183
Apologies and Appreciations ... 191
Spiral Healing ... 196
Ancestral Meditation ... 204

INTRODUCTION

We are the dreams of our ancestors. We carry their lives within our DNA and within our energy bodies. We carry both the shredded remnants of past wounds and the shining grain of sand that created the pearl. If we can inherit trauma, we can inherit strength and wisdom as well. Your ancestors can pass on their gifts, their blessings, and their wisdom through your dreams, and their pain, suffering, and trauma can get transmitted through your nightmares. Sometimes the pain of the past is more than can be transmuted in one lifetime. Sometimes the pearl and the pain have different origins.

Let's stop here for a minute to reflect: We are the dreams of our ancestors. Deep in your history, your ancestors—your parents, grandparents, great-grandparents, great-great-grandparents, as far back as you can imagine and then some—had a dream, an image, a vision of what they hoped for the lives of their descendants. *You* are that dream, the time-traveled embodiment of their hopes and visions. Therefore, ultimately, this is a book about healing and hope. You and your ancestors have been through wounding and trauma as well as freedom and redemption. As the psychologist Diana Fosha tells us, we are wired for healing.[1] So, the trajectory is ultimately that of attaching and connecting, moving forward, repairing, and blessing.

Think of a *matryoshka* doll. These Russian nesting dolls can also represent who you are and what you encompass: one doll nesting inside the other until you get to your core self. Dreams can take you into the heart of your healing. They help you go forward and backward in time to heal from

---

1. Fosha, "Wired for Healing."

Introduction

your personal, ancestral, and global wounds. Then, when combined with dream-guided action steps, you will pass on healing rather than wounding to the next generation.

Barack Obama titled his first book *Dreams from My Father: A Story of Race and Inheritance*. In the book, he discusses his multiracial and intergenerational inheritance. Obama wrote that for his grandparents, his admission into Punahou Academy (where he studied from fifth grade through high school graduation) heralded the start of something far-reaching and impressive. It represented an elevation in the family's status that they took great pains to share widely. With Obama's admission and eventual graduation, some of his ancestors got to see their dreams come true while they were still living.

Telling the stories of your ancestors and your family lets you know that you are a part of something larger than yourself alone, that your identity has connection and continuity in time and space. It connects you to the web of time and the web of life.

As you begin to tune in to your dreams, notice if your ancestors have been trying to contact you, either through shouts or whispers. Asleep or awake, is there a character or an animal that has been following you around lately, or for several years? This may be your ancestors whispering to you, "Listen. I am still here. Tracking. Watching. Communicating." Both the common themes and the reoccurring characters in your dreams can give you hints about their messages. For example, if you frequently dream that you are being chased: Are you being chased by someone or something, such as a large dog or monster? Who or what is *truly* chasing you? If there is fear involved in the chase, is that the equivalent of a shout desperately trying to get your intention? "Wait up, I have something for you!" or "I need you—help me!" or even "Watch out, this grudge is not resolved." Or are your ancestors whispering? These ancestors may be gentler, but they can still be persistent. Is it a gift they are trying to give you, or an offer or request for healing?

The Dream Journal

If you don't already have one, purchase a dream journal. This could be a beautiful hardcover journal or a simple spiral notebook. Your dream journal can be dedicated to your dreams only, or you can use it as a combination of journal writing, drawing, daytime thoughts and synchronicities, and records of your nighttime dreams—just be sure to differentiate between these types of writings so that you remember when and how you learned something.

Keep your dream journal by your bed so that you can begin (or continue) to capture the shouts and whispers that come to you through your dreams. Honor every fragment. No dream is unimportant. No dream is too small. A fragment can be worth a thousand words.

Write the date of each dream on the page. As you fill your dream journal, begin to take notice of common characters, objects, themes, or emotions from dream to dream. Notice the emotional story of the dream: Was it pleasant, unpleasant, or scary? You might take a highlighter and underline or circle the common elements between your dreams. Pay particular attention to dreams that contain family members, past or present. It's possible that people in your dreams will feel like family, even if they are not yet unidentifiable; make note of that too.

Ancestor Dreams

Recently, I have been having dreams about my ancestors. One vivid dream had to do with making borscht, a hearty Ukrainian beet soup often served with sour cream.

> *I am learning the borscht recipe from a chef. It seems that we needed a piece of equipment called a shredder to make the soup. The chef helps me locate one. After that, I am in charge of teaching my students how to do it. They aren't getting it right, so we have to start over from scratch now that we have the shredder.*

Since the dream, I have had a new craving for beets. I believe this dream is a message from my Ukrainian ancestors. My grandfather was born in Kiev, and around 1905, he and his family left the Ukraine to escape the pogroms at the turn of the century. Just as a dream has many layers, I wonder how else my ancestors' experiences affect me today. For example, when I walk alone on dark streets, my heart beats faster. How much of that is ancestral, a remnant of my ancestors' trauma? How much is neurobiological, with the brain's encoding for safety? How much is personal, a remnant of an attempted assault when I was in my twenties? How much is cultural, simply being a woman walking alone at night and the relative safety—or lack thereof—in our society?

The very fact that your ancestors survived, sometimes against all odds, is testament to the power of your ancestral dreams. Somewhere in your history, in the near or far past, ancestors whispered to their children, "Survive. Take this amulet, this sacred text, these beads, these words, these candlesticks, this recipe, this clod of earth, and carry our story onward."

Your history is not only passed on by your biological family, but by anyone who loved, parented, cared for, or influenced you. These individuals created a matrix that contains the seeds of their hopes and dreams for the next generation. The land itself holds memories, pain, and healing as well as the people who walk on it. There is an old Hebrew *midrash* (story or parable) that each blade of grass that springs forth from the earth has its own personal angel whispering to it, "Grow."

Recently, I met with my client Daniel, and we spoke about ancestors and legacies. We did some waking embodied dreamwork with the rocks, shells, and other bits of magical stuff I have in my office.[2] As he left, I walked out the door with him and scooped up a handful of earth from my garden. I pressed the earth into his hand and said, "Take this. Literal grounding. To hold and remember." We do not need to continue to carry the heaviest rocks anymore; the earth will help keep us grounded.

The Healing Journey

The purpose of this book is to help you connect with your ancestors in order to heal any intergenerational wounds you may have inherited, to receive the intergenerational blessings and wisdom gifted to you, and to pass on these healed and whole legacies to your children and your chil-

---

2. Waking embodied dreamwork is an integrated dreamwork approach that uses a variety of somatic, tactile, expressive, and kinesthetic approaches to engage with the dream. The dreamer uses all of their senses, their physical body, and their environment to gain a deeper understanding of the many possible layers in a dream. For example, a spiral shell on the mantle could represent the dream metaphor of "running in circles," presenting an opportunity to reframe that metaphor from a dream.

dren's children. A powerful way to do this is to tap into the consciousness of your dreams, both your sleep and waking dream states of reverie, trance, guided imagery, meditation, and synchronicity. You can do this with intentionality, with purpose, and with vision: to forgive, to repair, to connect, to heal, and to transmit. You can take your place in the line of your ancestors, knowing that the proverbial buck stops here.

Intergenerational trauma, also called *ancestral trauma* or *legacy burdens*, is a concept that is making its way into practices such as Internal Family Systems (IFS), Eye Movement Desensitization and Reprocessing (EMDR), developmental studies, somatic therapies, and Hellinger Constellation therapies. Ancestor healing is also receiving more public attention thanks to Black, Indigenous, and People of Color (BIPOC) traditional and indigenous communities. The Western world is only just starting to recognize what land-based and Eastern traditions have known for centuries: We have a responsibility to our ancestors and our descendants to offer healing and to accept their wisdom. If your ancestors have not been completely laid to rest, they can inhabit your nights and days. Your task is not only to offer healing to their spirits and send them back to the light, but to discern and differentiate between what is your own work and what is *not* part of you: not part of your own soul's mission, not yours to carry. I will return to this concept in more detail in subsequent chapters, for this discernment is a core part of the healing journey.

You have likely passed customs or habits on to your descendants through your parenting, your wisdom, your ideas, your gene pool, your energy field, and your very dreams or nightmares. Sometimes family members can even share dreams as well. One member of my dream circle, Mia, actually dreams her daughter's dreams some nights. Mia and her daughter frequently dream share in the morning and regularly find elements of their dreams—or even entire dreams—that are practically identical.

Nature, Nurture, or Both?

My wonderful daughter, who was adopted from China at a year old, frequently says that she inherited things from us (her parents) like a certain stoicism in the face of pain or a taste or distaste for certain foods. (For example, loving coffee ice cream from me, and an aversion to bananas from her dad.) She uses that word too: "inherited." Sometimes she is clear that she learned a value, an attitude, or a skill from us, saying, "That's because I have a therapist for a mom" or "I have a physical therapist for a dad." Other times the implication is that she did inherit that something in the traditional sense of the word. Is this nature, nurture, or a combination of both?

There is clearly an environmental influence, but my daughter also has a felt sense of inheriting things from our gene pool that she has no literal connection to, in addition to what she inherited in the more traditional sense of the word from her biological parents, grandparents, and ancestors. My daughter has inherited traits like compassion and persistence in the face of obstacles as well as deep connections with her grandparents (our parents) on both sides of the veil. She might be more correct than we know in this. After all, I sent her the red thread of energetic connection across time and space the moment we received the adoption paperwork that she was to be our daughter, known in adoption circles as "the referral." I maintained that red thread of energetic connection until I held her in my arms, and that process was about the length of time of a "traditional" pregnancy. The opening sentence of my first book on dreams, *Modern Dreamwork*, is: "Twenty years ago I dreamed my daughter home."[3] Our energetic genes combined with her biological genes across time and space to create our family.

Tracked By Our Old Dreams

About twenty years ago, I had the following dream.

> *I am in the desert, leading a long line of women undulating and snaking our way over the sand dunes to answer the call of the drumming coming from a large, low tent. As we approach and then enter the tent, I see the female drummers seated in the center, and the rest of us make our way around them to join in the ceremony.*

Fast forward to an International Association for the Study of Dreams (IASD) conference I attended in 2023. In a workshop, I was inspired by others to bring this dream forward to explore with the group. It still

---

3. Schiller, *Modern Dreamwork*, 1.

Introduction

haunted me, and it still had resonance, so I knew that I wasn't done with it yet. What was my inheritance in this dream? What drum call did I have yet to answer for myself, my ancestors, and my descendants? What was the message from my ancestors that I was supposed to pass on? I knew there were more rituals and ceremonies that I must continue to partake in.

The following year, I attended the 2024 IASD conference, and a harvest festival coincided with the dates of the conference. A group of women spontaneously created a ceremony to honor our ancestors and the land. We gathered with homemade drums, fruit and wine, and song and dance. We erected a canopy of sacred blue light to honor the harvest festival. I get shivers as I reread this—it feels like part of my old dream coming to life.

Guided and interactive dreamwork, as well as dreamwork within a group, can enhance your ability to dream through the healing that you, your family, the world, and the land so need. Not only are two heads better than one, but a group of heads and hearts can enter the dream space together and enlarge the vision and the learnings. When you connect with others in shared humanity and the conjoint power found in deep meditation, prayer, energy work, and dreamwork, the result is greater than the sum of its parts. Your dreams are your own sacred text, your personal road map, that can connect you with sacred scriptures of your own heritage.

The dream I had was connected, at least in part, to bringing ways of feminine knowledge and wisdom traditions forward. Bringing forth dreamwork, ritual, and ceremony is not necessarily linear or logical. Somehow, this dream connected me with my roots, those in the Ukraine, the Netherlands, Austria, and the Middle East specifically. The desert has always spoken loudly to me across time and space.

Noted dreamer, shamanic practitioner, and author Robert Moss teaches that there are threefold paths of the ancestors: the ancestors of your bloodlines, of the lands where you live and travel, and of your spiritual lineages. The land itself is an ancestor too—Gaia herself, the living sentient land—all the way back to the origin stories of most world traditions.

We know that unresolved issues from an individual's or collective's past can become their destiny.[4] The past tends to repeat itself until we have

---

4. Hübl, *Healing Collective Trauma.*

the courage to face it together. Story coach and somatic writing developer Tanya Taylor Rubinstein continues this thread forward: Each of us can become a great ancestor for our future lineage. In doing so, you will not only heal your own ancestral line but also contribute to the healing of humanity. One of my dream circle friends is named Marcia. One day, the group examined a dream of hers that included her deceased mom as well as her daughter and new granddaughter. Afterward, Marcia told us that she felt even more of a responsibility to be a good ancestor.

You can reach out to your ancestors in your dreams. This usually refers to departed ancestors, but as we have expanded the meaning of the word, you can also reach out to the land and to your actual or potential descendants now and in the future. You can pray or direct thoughts and intentions to general or specific ancestors. If you send healing to all your relations, who comes through to you? You may encounter the known or the unknown: a lineage you were aware of, or a past that you did not yet know of consciously.

Working with others to complete an uncompleted action as indicated by your dream adds the glue of connection to the healing process. Healing ripples forward and backward in time, to your ancestors and to your descendants. Soul energy is not bound by time or space, so when you heal an ancestral soul wound, the love and compassion and forgiveness that you give to yourself or to others can echo throughout generations. It is always "now" in a dreamscape, never yesterday or tomorrow. Likewise, it is always now in sacred time as well as the time of the soul.

What to Expect

In chapter 1, I will examine the six calls your ancestors may be using to try to get through to you, via both shouts and whispers:

1. "I am still here, and you are not alone."
2. "Take these gifts, blessings, or apologies."
3. "Let me help, heal, or warn you."
4. "Please, please help and heal me; I am still suffering."
5. "Watch out: This old grudge has not yet been resolved."

Introduction

6. "Carry on my name and gifts to your children and your children's children. Remember."

I will also examine the continuum of consciousness and how the shouts and whispers of your ancestors may come through at any of these levels.

Chapter 2 will explore the literal, metaphorical, and spiritual meanings of bones, marrow, and stem cells in dreamwork and in relationship to your ancestors. I will share some of the links between life and afterlife that we can learn by examining our bone memories.

Chapter 3 will explore epigenetics, how the DNA strands of previous generations get passed down to us, and how events in the lives of your ancestors can affect your very DNA through a process called *methylation*.

Chapter 4 looks at how the relationship between ancestors and dream messages is considered in several traditions. This chapter also explores the unique circumstances of ancestry and adoption.

Chapter 5 will examine the nature of grieving you may have with various ancestors. Grief has many forms: You may have simple or complicated grief. You may miss some beloveds greatly, or just a little. You may be relieved someone is gone. You may have never met the ancestor who has passed. All this and more influences your relationship with your ancestors. Things that can help you find closure and peace will be addressed here.

Chapter 6 will provide an overview of some current body-based trauma treatments as they relate to ancestral work. The nature of inherited and embodied trauma for yourself and your ancestors will be examined, and I will discuss healing body, mind, heart, and spirit through ancestral waking and sleeping dreamwork.

Chapter 7 outlines the GAIA method, the Guided Active Imagination Approach I have developed. The GAIA method forms one of the cornerstones of safe, interactive dreamwork with nightmares and bad dreams. I will also share how to apply this method to intergenerational trauma and healing.

Chapters 8, 9, and 10 will provide a deeper dive into additional methods, resources, rituals, and dreamwork for healing intergenerational traumas, honoring the ancestors, and accessing your legacy gifts.

Each chapter includes multiple exercises that allow you to follow by example, practice on your own, and heal from within.

EXERCISE
Building Your Genogram

A genogram is a pictorial representation of a family tree. Your genogram will allow you to keep track of who's who in your family, and you may see familial patterns in this visual format. I recommend referencing the image provided here to create your own genogram. If you prefer to make a genogram digitally, there are many templates online that you can use.

1. Begin by drawing a symbol for yourself. Typically, squares represent men and circles represent women, though there are numerous other identity symbols that can be found online. Symbols can also be adapted to fit your needs so long as the meaning is clear to you.

2. Once you have drawn yourself, incorporate other generations of your family. If family members are older than you, they will go above your symbol, while younger generations members will come below. Members of the same generation should be parallel to each other. Here are some other basic genogram tips:

   - Partnered couples are linked with a horizontal line. A slash on the horizontal line between two parents indicates a divorce or separation. A dotted horizontal line represents the parties are partnered but not married.

   - Offspring are connected via vertical lines that extend from the horizontal line linking their parents.

   - An X over a square or circle indicates the individual is deceased.

   - A triangle indicates an impending birth or unknown gender. If there is an X over the triangle, it indicates a miscarriage or stillbirth.

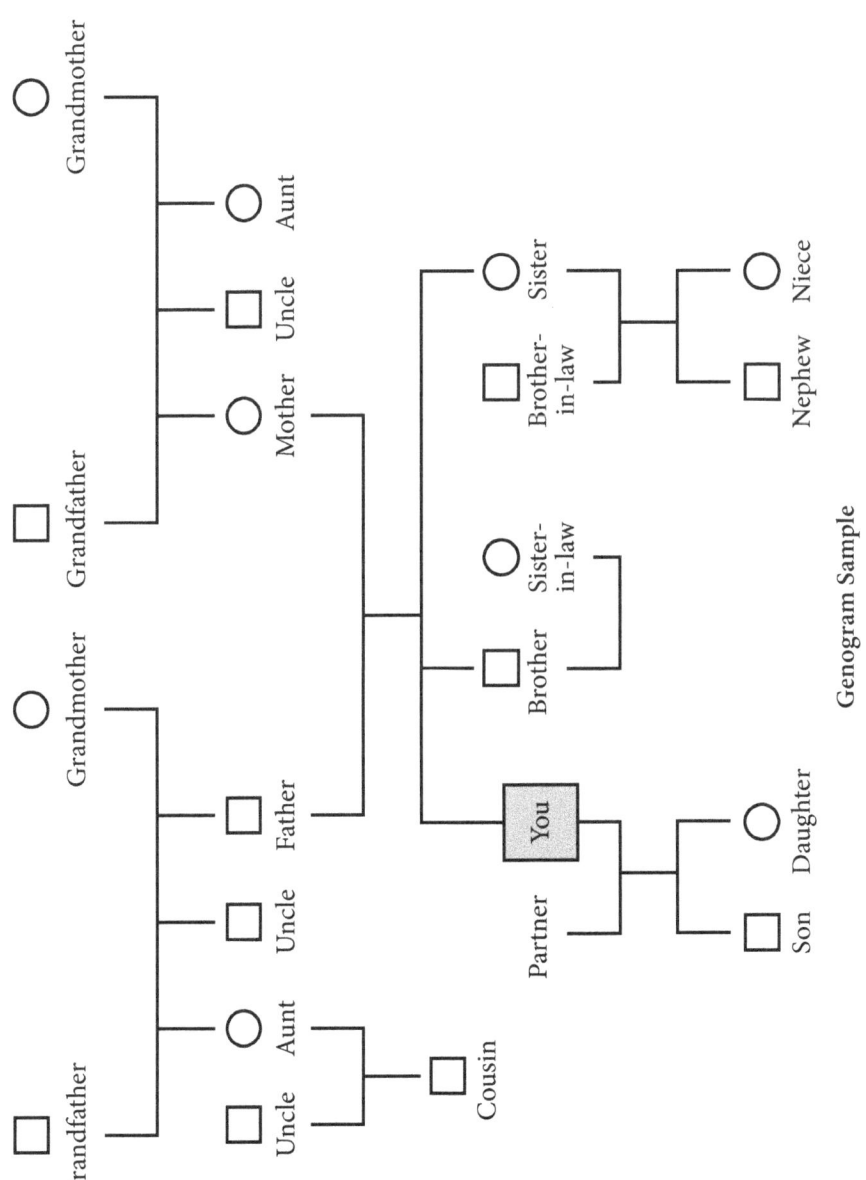

Genogram Sample

3. As you link symbols on your genogram, write in the names and ages of family members. If a family member was adopted, write in the age they were when they were adopted and where they were adopted from. Add death dates and causes of death for family members who are no longer alive. See how many generations of your family tree you can represent in your genogram, including countries of origin as far back as you can.

4. Then, take your genogram a step further by adding any relevant information underneath family member's names. For example, you may wish to write their profession, existing medical conditions, mental health history, history of traumatic events, or special skills or gifts.

As you make your way through this book, you will be able to add even more information to your genogram, which will help you see the patterns in your family tree more clearly. Return to your genogram to fill out your ancestral history as it emerges.

ONE

WHAT ARE YOUR ANCESTORS TELLING YOU OR ASKING OF YOU?

> A family is essentially a field of stories, each intricately connected. Death does not sever the connection; rather, the story expands as it continues unwinding inter-dimensionally....According to the Old Ones...time is a weave, a DNA spiral moving within, through us, and around us. It is always changing.
> —*Joy Harjo,* Poet Warrior

How do your ancestors get your attention: through shouts or through whispers? By way of your dreams or nightmares, or in your waking life? Both Buddhist philosophy and a children's nursery rhyme tell us that "life is but a dream." For some dreams, we are asleep, and for others we are awake: Waking dreams include noticing signs we may have missed before, including uncanny coincidences, déjà vu, and prescient experiences of knowing something before it happens.

Your ancestors may come to you unasked, or you may intentionally call or invoke them; we will look at both sides of this coin in this chapter. When you do hear from your ancestors, they may whisper so softly that you need to stop, tune in, and pay attention to hear them, or they may shout so loudly—especially if they are showing up in your nightmares—that your natural tendency is to intentionally avoid their messages, almost like putting your fingers in your ears and saying, "La, la, la" so as not to hear. These messages can be intense; I don't blame you. But your ancestors' messages won't go away until you stop and listen so that you can respond to their request.

Chapter One

According to a 2023 study, 53 percent of Americans report connections with their ancestors who have departed, most of them through their dreams.[5] In addition to dream visits and connections, some reported hearing their ancestor's voice inside their head while awake. Others experienced a "felt sense" in their bodies. These connections are sometimes simply a felt presence of the ancestor in the room or vicinity. Sometimes our ancestors show up as themselves in our dreams, and sometimes they are symbolized, hidden, or disguised as metaphor. In that case, we must then decode their messages and true identities.

Connections with your ancestors can come through any of your senses and may involve words, emotions, images, or an experiential knowing. You are likely already connected with some of your ancestral legacy, but one of the signs of deep work in the spiritual or energetic realm is the "aha" of a surprise, the frisson of an embodied knowing: "Oh, I didn't know that before" or "I sort of knew that, but I wasn't sure until now."

As you will see in this chapter, you may receive messages from your ancestors during any of the states of consciousness.

The Continuum of Consciousness

We all experience a continuum of consciousness that ranges from wide awake to sound asleep and beyond. Held within these end points are the in-between states in which we have access to other ways of knowing.

In the first five stages, from wide awake to chemically altered, we retain various levels of consciousness or awareness with the waking world. These are in the states in which you may have waking dreamish experiences, known as uncanny coincidences or, in Jungian terms, synchronicities. It has also been called a "glitch in the matrix" of waking consciousness.

The middle stage of the hypnopompic or hypnogogic zones refer to being in-between waking and sleeping, either as you are falling asleep or as you gradually awaken. In the hypnopompic and hypnogogic zones, you retain a dual awareness of both the waking and sleeping worlds. Don't neglect what comes through to you in these in-between states, where the

---

5. Tevington and Corichi, "Many Americans Report Interacting with Dead Relatives in Dreams or Other Ways."

veil between worlds is thinner. These images and scenes are dreams too, and they can be unpacked just as a dream can be. In other words, a dream in this in-between state is still a dream.

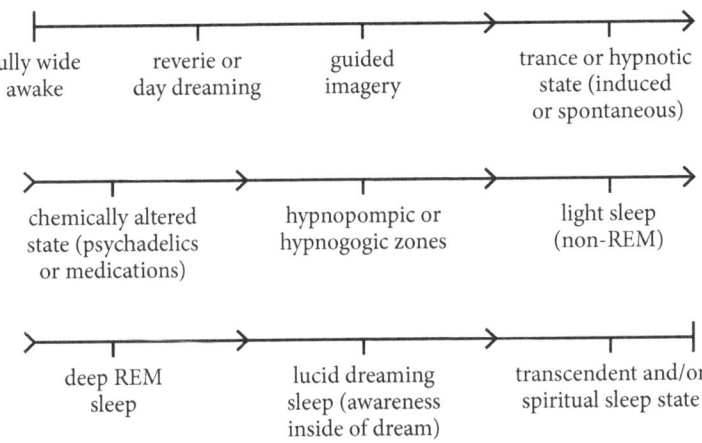

Continuum of Consciousness

In the deeper stages of sleep, we do not retain active awareness of what is happening in the outside world unless it permeates the dream world in some unusual way. For example, I once dreamt that I was in an earthquake, an unusual dream for me. When I awoke, I discovered that a jackhammer was tearing up the street in front of my house, and the sound and vibration had permeated my waking/sleep barrier in symbolic form as an earthquake.

Lucid dreaming has its own unique place in dreams. In this state, the individual is sound asleep and dreaming, but at the same time, they are aware they are having a dream. This skill can be acquired with practice; I recommend researching lucid dreaming exercises. Lucid dreaming can also happen spontaneously.

We move in and through endless spirals of time and place, not only in a straight line from past to future, which is easier for us to picture, but also in spirals that are contained within us. When the veil between worlds is thinner—either because of grief or loss, or because you are straddling the threshold of waking and sleeping—you can more easily access your departed loved ones and any resources you may need to heal and finish their journeys.

Another example of in-betweenness was when my friend Bob's father died but had not yet been buried. Bob described to me his in-between state of feeling like time had stopped, that he was treading water, and the ongoing connection with his dad felt fragile and fuzzy. Still there, and yet not there. He anticipated a greater clarity once his father's body was buried and it was "clearer" as to which world he was in. His dad was between worlds in multiple senses of meaning. I agreed with Bob that the clarity in their relationship would return once his dad was "settled" into his new reality.

The Six Ancestral Calls

I have identified six types of messages that people tend to receive from their ancestors.

1. "I am still here, and you are not alone."
2. "Take these gifts, blessings, or apologies."
3. "Let me help, heal, or warn you."
4. "Please, please help and heal me; I am still suffering."
5. "Watch out: This old grudge has not yet been resolved."
6. "Carry on my name and gifts to your children and your children's children. Remember."

Remember that messages may come through in multiple layers of consciousness including while asleep, while in reverie states, or out-of-the-blue in waking consciousness. Each type of call, be it a shout or a whisper, may require a different kind of response. Some of these calls ask that we listen and respond, others ask us to do something, and still others make demands.

The Blue Container of Safety and Light

Before you go any further, I want to teach you how to create a safe and protective container in which you can explore your ancestors' shouts and whispers. This is essential for safe, effective dreamwork.

What Are Your Ancestors Telling You or Asking of You?

Some of your ancestral connections will be lovely blessings full of guidance. Some will be difficult, painful, or heartbreaking. Whether you know or suspect that your ancestors are still hurting, whether you fear they may hurt you in some way, or just for good, protected dreamwork, create a container of safety and light. Then, you will be better protected from the shouts and hear the whispers more clearly.

Dreams are made in large part from energy, and energy is made from light. Ancestral beings are part of this light. We come from light before we are born and return to it after death. When you dream, you may travel to realms you can't access while awake and may even have encounters with ancestors in this liminal space. That is why it is important to create a container of safety and light before beginning dreamwork.

To create your container, begin by visualizing a blue light. Lucid dreamers advise us to look for the blue light when we feel that we are surrounded by darkness or are in the void. The color blue indicates that we are protected, loved, and seen and has numerous spiritual connotations throughout history.[6] For millennia, deities have been depicted with blue faces, and Jesus's mother Mary was clothed in blue and white robes. Colette Aboulker-Muscat, the pioneer of Kabbalistic dreamwork, focused on the healing power of dreams and dream imagery, and she believed sapphire was the color of spirit and should be used especially for dreaming, visioning, and guided imagery. Colette and her student Catherine Shainberg created a version of the following exercise to keep readers safe and grounded while exploring other realms and connecting with those beyond this time and place.[7]

EXERCISE
Creating a Sapphire-Blue Container of Light

I encourage you to intentionally create a container of light any time you are going to be delving into deep dreamwork or connecting with your ancestors. Always use this method when connecting with or calling upon ancestors who are in pain, ancestors

---

6. Johnson, *Llewellyn's Complete Book of Lucid Dreaming*; Waggoner, *Lucid Dreaming*.
7. Shainberg, *The Kabbalah of Light*, xviii, 9, 87.

who are struggling, or ancestors who want something from you. This method will help you keep your boundaries intact as you do your work. Eventually, you can share your blue light container with ancestors who need healing when the time comes.

1. Quiet your body and mind. Plant your feet on the ground, barefoot if possible. In this moment, you are connecting with your first ancestor, Mother Earth.

2. Close your eyes and imagine a line coming down from the heavens, through the crown of your head, and down through your body. Ground this plumb line through the soles of your feet into the earth, connecting above and below. Bring awareness of your body into the present with your breathing.

3. Next, take a deep breath through your nose, inhaling slowly to the count of four. Exhale slowly to the count of eight through your mouth, pursing your lips like you are blowing out candles on a birthday cake. Do this three times to put yourself into a light trance state.

4. Then, visualize and feel yourself surrounded by an egg-shaped container of sapphire light. If this color doesn't work for you, find the color and shade of safety and protection that feels just right. Your blue light may come through as turquoise, sapphire, teal, aquamarine, azure, opalescent, or crystal blue. Let yourself be enveloped by this light.

Message One: "I Am Still Here, and You Are Not Alone."

Perhaps the most ubiquitous message from the ancestors is that the connection across time and space does not end with death. Cultures and traditions around the globe have spoken with, honored, and connected with their dearly departed. For example, on *Día de los Muertos* ("Day of the Dead") in Mexico, some families have picnics in graveyards to honor and spend time with the ancestors. In China, many homes have an altar dedicated to their ancestors in a place of honor in the home; the ancestors may be offered food and drink. At Jewish cemeteries, small stones are placed on graves as physical signs that they have been visited by loved ones. The ancestors talk to us too, via words or signs or dreams.

One of the most comforting dreams to have after the loss of a loved one is a visitation dream. There is a vividness, a numinous quality to these dream visits that is qualitatively different than a dream about the relative. A dream about a relative may be something like "My mom was a character in my dream last night" or "There was a woman with red hair who was not really my mom but was my mother in the dream." However, a dream visitation often includes a felt sense of the spirit of the departed. Many dreamers hear their loved one's voice as if in real time, feel their touch, or sense their presence in a way that is immensely comforting. It is as if their loved one is saying, "I am here. You are not alone."

When my client Ellen's beloved cat died, she told me that she woke from a dream feeling him sitting right on her chest, purring. Margarite said that she turned in her dream-sleep and felt her deceased husband gently kiss her cheek. My friend Gwen's sister has dreamt of their departed mother every night for over thirty years; it is a comfort to her. Shaman and dreamer Robert Moss states that not only do we dream of our departed, but they dream of us as well, and they try to reach us through our dreams.[8] The message or information they have for us can vary, hence the different types of callings.

Twenty-plus years after his death, my stepfather Bud is still very present for me. I hear his voice when I ask him a question in my waking dreamtime, and sometimes spontaneously in a nighttime dream as well. Since his death, we've joked that he married my mom both to be her husband and because he was meant to be a mentor and wisdom guide for me. He was my first reader for all my professional articles when I taught at Boston University (he was a professor himself) and was full of life and light.

For some reason, my stepfather Bud has the ability to traverse the veil between worlds with me more easily than my other ancestors. Perhaps it has to do with the fact that I was with him at the hospital in his final days. He could communicate with us only by blinking his eyes purposefully

---

8. Moss, "Dreaming with the Departed."

when we asked him to let us know that he could hear us or asked if he was enjoying our singing to him. In this way, Bud and I established a nonverbal and unordinary form of communication before he passed on, when he was on the threshold between worlds. I was blessed to be able to say goodbye one final time just hours before he died, and I remember encouraging him to let go. As I reflect on our continued connection, this explanation for his availability even after death feels right.

Message Two: "Take These Gifts, Blessings, or Apologies."

Gifts and blessings can come from your ancestors in many ways. They may come in the form of a gesture, an object, in words, or in actions. When you make an ongoing place for your ancestors in your life, you are more likely to notice their offerings.

In your dreams, have you noticed a figure that seems numinous in some way? Perhaps they were glowing or larger than life. Whether you recognized the figure as a relative or not, they may have been an ancestor showing up with a gift or blessing for you. Sometimes dreams make it quite clear that a gift is being offered; other times, you may need to unpack and explore the dream to find a gift.

My colleague Gabrielle was diagnosed with breast cancer for the second time at the start of the COVID-19 pandemic. I can only imagine how difficult that must have been, especially given the isolation many of us struggled with during the pandemic. In addition to receiving medical care, Gabrielle prayed and dreamed for her healing. She told me that one morning she woke up feeling the loving presence of her ancestors nearby. Gabrielle's ancestors accompanied her through the dream state, into the hypnopompic in-between zone, and then into her waking state, and they offered her an additional name: Ariella, which means "Lioness of God." Having the loving support of her ancestors helped Gabrielle on her journey, and she began to live up to new soul-name. Gabrielle, which means "Strength of God," infused her given name with her new Lioness self. Her name-gift of Lioness-Strength was a powerful gift from her ancestors that helped her through as she joined her present and her future. It was the beginning of a spiritual journey that continues to this day—Gabrielle recently celebrated her four-year anniversary of being cancer-free.

Josh dreamed that Spock from *Star Trek* showed up in his dream and made the Vulcan salute with his hands, which means "live long and prosper." This gesture had special meaning for Josh, as he knew it to be a blessing—the inspiration for this gesture was a Hebrew benediction. Leonard Nimoy (the actor who played Spock) was born in Boston, but his parents were from a village in the Ukraine. As a boy, Nimoy attended a service at an Orthodox Jewish Synagogue and witnessed a rabbi using this symbol to bless the congregation. Years later, when Nimoy felt that his character, Spock, needed to make a "greeting gesture," he chose the gesture he had seen at the synagogue about twenty-five years prior.[9] The Vulcan salute went on to become a gesture associated with *Star Trek*, but Nimoy never forgot its origins. "This is the shape of the letter shin," Nimoy said in a 2013 interview, making the famous Vulcan salute.[10] The Hebrew letter shin, he noted, is the first letter in several Hebrew words, including *Shaddai* (a name for God), *shalom* (the word for hello, goodbye, and peace) and *Shechinah*, the feminine aspect of God, the indwelling presence. Josh, who grew up Jewish, immediately resonated with this blessing, as his relatives too were originally from the Ukraine, and as a big sci-fi fan, he had lived with Mr. Spock since his childhood.

Sometimes, however, a dream's gift or blessing is less obvious. It may be disguised as something or someone chasing you, or as a warning of impending danger of some sort. Your initial response might to be run and hide instead of to receive. But once you are safe and protected within the dream itself (or afterward, in your waking dreamwork), you can then discover what the blessing or gift is. We will talk more about how to do this in chapter 7.

My friend Molly told me about a powerful dream her grandmother Ruchel had while she was a prisoner in a Nazi concentration camp. Ruchel still planned to fast for Yom Kippur, the fasting day of atonement, when prayers asking for forgiveness and a fresh start in the new year are said.

---

9. Nimoy, "How Leonard Nimoy's Jewish Roots Inspired the Vulcan Salute."
10. Ohlheiser, "The Jewish Roots of Leonard Nimoy and 'Live Long and Prosper.'"

Chapter One

The night before the fast, Ruchel had a dream in which she experienced a very clear visit from her departed grandfather. He said to her, "Don't fast! You are already starving, and you need to survive. Eat as much as you can every day and survive this place. Live." Ruchel followed her grandfather's instructions and ate the next day. She survived, and now her descendants include children, grandchildren, and great-grandchildren. Following her ancestor's guidance aided not only Ruchel's own survival, it ensured the survival of her family line as well.

Ancestral gifts can also be hidden inside a nightmare. In my book *PTSDreams*, Dina had a nightmare in which she was being chased by a giant around an old-fashioned village.[11] At one point in the dream, Dina heard a voice advising her to turn around and look into the eyes of the giant. When she did, she found that rather than being threatening, his eyes were kind, and then the giant picked her up and danced with her. The dream that began as a nightmare shifted, and it ended with Dina feeling relieved and safe.

When I revisit this dream now in the context of ancestral blessings and gifts, I find new meaning. Dina's ancestors escaped the Holocaust in Eastern Europe. She is alive today because her family members escaped a truly terrifying real-world giant. Growing up in America in the fifties and sixties, Dina and her siblings did not have to run for their lives, but Dina inherited the intense felt-sense memories of her mother and other family members who felt distress, fear, and panic.

The ancestral gifts in Dina's dream showed up in two ways: One, this dream was a message to stop and listen to the Voice when it spoke to her, and two, it was a reminder to dance. Even inside the dream, Dina was able to stop and listen to the Divine Voice advising her that she didn't need to run from this giant. Rather, the Voice conveyed that it was safe for Dina to stop and dance with this larger-than-life being.

Today, Dina is both a spiritual director and a dance choreographer. Her most recent choreography vividly depicts her mother's journey from the dangers across the Atlantic to safer harbors in the new world. At age ninety, her mother was in the audience during the debut performance. Addition-

---

11. Schiller, *PTSDreams*, 89.

ally, Dina just performed in a multimedia dance and performance-art piece on grief and healing called "Under the Canopy." When we join in community under the canopy of our shared grief and are wrapped in love, we heal. Dina's gifts keep going forward and backward in time.

A dream's gift or blessing may also be in the form of a long-awaited apology. Your ancestor may have passed before you reconciled your differences, which could leave you feeling cut off or angry at words that were said or actions that were taken. The gift in this message might be a healing apology or making amends, and it can go both ways. You can make peace with the departed even after they have gone, so don't neglect this opportunity. You can finish up your unfinished business on the other side of the veil if necessary. It is never too late to say, "I'm sorry. I forgive you. I do love you." Once you understand the context for another's actions, including the hurtful ones, through your own healing work, it is easier to have compassion for them and their missteps in life.

Message Three: "Let Me Help, Heal, or Warn You."

In this type of message, your ancestors are actively trying to get a message to you in order to help you or warn you of something. Are you listening? Sometimes, these messages are hidden in dreams that feel negative or scary; a hurt or needy ancestor may be aggressive in their requests or demands. In many cases, this message is intense because it is your ancestor's way of grabbing your attention. Particularly if you are confused or struggling with a dilemma in your life, they may simply be trying to help or offer advice.

Are you the type who is easily receptive to offers of assistance, or are you a loner, an "I can do it myself, thank you very much" type? Although I am not a loner, when I was in my twenties I had to learn how to say "Yes, thank you" when I was offered help. One incident has stuck with me: While my then-boyfriend was over at my house, my roommate offered to help me with something. I declined her offer because I didn't really need the help. My boyfriend said to me, "Yael, she wants to help you. Don't deny her the gift of helping, whether you really require it or not." This was an important life lesson for me, as the daughter of a single mother who was taught the importance of being independent.

Chapter One

What does it take to get your attention or for you to accept an offer of help? For some, this is not a problem at all; they easily accept and simply say thank you when help is offered. However, if you have a difficult time asking for and receiving help, chances are that you have been frequented by a figure—known or unknown—in your dreams for quite some time. In these dreams, an ancestor, a power animal, or a divine being will show up. You can tune in to this dream figure and ask them what message they have, or once you have woken up, you can reflect on this in your journal by asking, "What did they come to tell me or help me with?" See what answers you can find. Perhaps you have already identified an area of your life where you need advice or assistance, or you may have a vague sense of something not quite right that your ancestors could help with.

Parents, particularly of teens or young adults, know that our kiddos would rather accept advice from almost anyone else. This potential tug of war is a normal, albeit infuriating, developmental stage. Luckily for them and for us, we can direct them to ask their dreams or grandparents (alive or dead) what they advise. In my experience, it's as good as nocturnal therapy—and free to boot! In my house, when my daughter has a dilemma that I can't really help her with, or when I don't want to be the one making the decision on her behalf, or when she has already ignored my advice, I suggest that she ask her grandmothers. She was close with both of them. At this point in time, both have died. My daughter will ask her grandmothers for assistance or dream on the dilemma, known as dream incubation; sometimes I think she just channels. Afterward, she frequently tells me who advised her: Gramma Inez or Gramma Mimi. I love that this is second nature in my home. Sometimes both of her grandmothers give her the same advice, and they really do give her sound advice that I can get behind! Where does the advice actually come from? In the end, it doesn't matter; my daughter gets to have self-agency, figure things out, and connect with her grandmothers in the process.

Sometimes departed loved ones send messages with multilayered meanings. My client Jennie's brother died a few years ago after a long struggle with substance abuse. He left behind a five-year-old child, Tommy. Tommy's mother could not reliably care for him, so recently Jennie was granted official custody of her nephew. A few days later, she had this dream.

What Are Your Ancestors Telling You or Asking of You?

My brother shows up in my dream and says to me, "I love you."

I say back to him, "What are you doing? You don't usually get all mushy like this."

He replies, "If I tell you that I love you, then you have to say it back to me, and then I get to hear you say it to me too."

Wow. After a short discussion, we both agreed that this was a visit; it had all the vividness and immediacy associated with a visitation. We talked about how this healing of spoken love—which all too often went unspoken in her family—goes forward and backward in time and space. It healed her brother, who needed to both speak love and hear it; to Jennie, who received the visit and the message; and on to the next generation. When Jennie shared the dream with Tommy, he replied, "That's my dad. Tell him I love him too."

This dream carried the message "Let me help/heal you," when an ancestor asks for help in their own healing or shares messages that can be passed down to our descendants.

Departed loved ones can also offer some very concrete advice. Julie's father died over ten years ago, but he remained a vital presence in her life. She spoke with him regularly and felt comforted and warmed by his presence. One day, Julie's mother began having terrible headaches. Julie took her to doctor after doctor, where she had scan after scan and tried multiple medications, all to no avail. Julie began to despair about finding a solution to her mother's chronic pain. One day, she left her mother in the bedroom, went into the kitchen, and called out to her father in frustration, asking him for any wisdom or guidance he could offer. She underscored the importance of the message by saying to him, "And I need it to be crystal clear. And really, really soon." Seconds later, her mother crept out of the bedroom, leaned against the doorjamb, and asked, "Do you think it could be my eyes?" Her father answered Julie's plea for help through her mother, the one who needed the help, clear as a bell and within seconds.

Julie realized that the one doctor she had not yet thought to consult was an ophthalmologist. She made an appointment for her mother as soon as possible. After the examination, the doctor said, "Most of the time I don't see people with this condition until after they are already blind.

You caught it just in time." Julie's mother had some type of inflammation pressing on nerves connected to her eyes, and this was causing the terrible headaches. A regiment of strong anti-inflammatory medication was prescribed, and the headaches resolved. Julie's mother retained her eyesight until her death several years later.

Message Four: "Please, Please Help and Heal Me; I Am Still Suffering."

This message means the ancestors need something from us. They suffered in some way and left something undone, unresolved, or unhealed when they died. Therefore, they were not able to complete their journey to the other side of the veil in peace. If you consider intergenerational trauma—trauma that is passed down from generation to generation—this is also the realm of unfinished business, loss, old hurts, and wounds that you may be carrying that are not actually your own. The pleas or cries for help may come to you in your dreams in the form of repetitive images or themes. These may be themes of being chased, suffering, feeling trapped, or being trapped. There may be cutoffs or family disconnections that have long outlived their original source. Ancestors may show up in your dreams or your life with heartbreaking requests or pleas, beseeching demands, and even threats: "You are my last chance. You have to help me. If you don't, I will curse you…" Always take extra care when engaging with these ancestors.

Whether those in your dreams are known or unknown to you, a first step is to ask yourself who they are in your life. Are they a relative that you recognize or a character that is representing a relative? Are there patterns in your dreams (or in your waking life, for that matter) that are unhealthy, that interfere with you leading a peaceful and well-connected life? These patterns can permeate both your waking and sleeping life.

If you are carrying something that is not actually from your own life, your ancestors may ask for or demand some form of resolution from the other side of the veil. These may be the shouts like "Help me! I am hurting! I am still trapped!" Ancestral wounds, also known as family legacy burdens in Internal Family Systems therapy, can be passed down from generation to generation until someone recognizes, names, and takes action to stop and change the pattern. I will teach you how to release these souls as part of your dreamwork.

You may be hearing the cries of pain and suffering from ancestors who were enslaved, victimized, displaced, marginalized, wounded, or massacred. You may be getting the guilt or self-righteousness from those who oppressed others. One member of my dream circle, Samantha, had ancestors who were enslavers in the South before the Civil War. For quite some time, her dreams contained themes of making amends for the actions of her grandparents and great-grandparents. These themes usually showed up as metaphor: One dream contained images from the game Go, with its little black and white pieces; another dream showcased the zodiac sign Libra holding the scales of justice. Samantha's dream-to-life action steps involved becoming an activist for social justice causes. Eventually, the dreams ceased as Samantha worked to balance the scales in her daily life.

Ancestral shouts and whispers can enter your awareness through dreams, language patterns, relationship styles, and synchronicities and uncanny coincidences in daily life. Even after you recognize them for what they are, these dreams can continue to haunt you until you have taken some steps to heal the legacies of pain, fear, abandonment, or suffering. The good news is that even if the source of the nightmare isn't your own life, you can be part of the healing trajectory for both your ancestors and your descendants. Rather than passing on trauma, you can pass on healing.

My colleague David had several dreams set in Bolechow, a city in the Ukraine that his ancestors emigrated from. The series of dreams took place over a four-year span, all connected to the pogroms and the Nazi Holocaust his ancestors survived. In the following dream, even though David himself is injured, he helps a woman in need, most likely a great-great-grandmother.

> *My right leg is hurt, but not bad. I have a bit of a limp. I have crutches that belong to a childhood friend. At first, they are too tall for me, but I adjust the angle of them and then they work. They even seem to shrink to my height after this. I am on a terrace overlooking a square—a courtyard. It is Bolechow as I have seen it recently on a visit.*

Chapter One

There are some stairs in front of me. They are solid, like concrete/metal stairs that are open in the back. I hear that a woman up there needs help. I forget about my bad leg and quickly run up there. With me now is another woman and two men, plus the woman that needs help.

The woman that needs help is very large. She has shoulder-length blonde hair. She needs to be carried down. I know how to do this, though I need someone on the other side of her. I reach my right arm around her neck and my left arm under her left knee. With another man on the other side doing the same, we can carry her without too much difficulty. They may be paramedics, and I act like them, knowing what to do. I think at least three of us end up carrying her, which is a little awkward, but I'm in a good position. Then we find out there is an elevator, so we don't have to carry her down the stairs.

I am now carrying the woman outside with one of the men. We walk toward an open, flat, hard-packed dirt area that has fences around it. It is some sort of international military place, which I assume has medical staff and equipment. There are two guards that look like a combination of police officers and soldiers. The one in charge tells us to put the woman down. The other(s) quickly set her down, but I gently lay her head down on the ground before stepping aside.

Some central elements in this dream include the setting, the characters, and the goal of helping the injured. The dream is set in Bolechow, a city David's ancestors lived in. David himself is injured, but he quickly rallies to help someone else in need—an archetypal wounded healer motif. David's own assistive devices, the crutches, magically conform to his needs so that he can carry on with his mission. He goes upstairs to help the injured woman. The word *up* can have many associations, depending on the dreamer, but one can be up to other realms, beyond the veil that separates worlds. David can't do it alone, however, and several allies assist him, a community of caregivers. His dreaming self even supplied him with paramedics!

The injured woman is large. Perhaps this blonde from the Ukraine is a symbol of the large number of relatives David lost in the pogroms? They succeed in getting her out (out of the building, out of the country) and take her somewhere she can get medical care. I find it noteworthy that at the end of the dream, David gently lowers the woman's head, providing care and compassion at the end of his time with her.

After about four years of these kinds of dreams, it seemed that David had resolved his family history sufficiently through his own dreamwork and personal healing, and he gave and received healing to his ancestors who suffered. His dreams then shifted. David began to dream about other massive traumas of death and displacement, including the Rwandan genocide and the genocide of Indigenous peoples. It seems that David's soul has chosen or been chosen for this as part of his life mission. He has since written about and lectured on these dream patterns.

Message Five: "Watch Out: This Old Grudge Has Not Yet Been Resolved."

When this dream message comes through, you may want to set some extra boundaries and take extra protections so that you don't take on the negative energies of the ancestor looking for revenge. Remember, their vendetta or grudge is not yours, but you may be needed to help resolve it so everyone can move on. If an angry ancestor comes through in your waking or sleeping dreamtime, I recommend doubling the strength or thickness of your blue container of light, adding an additional color or colors, and adding the Boundary Balance of tapping on your sternum as you invoke protection. Chapter 8 has a detailed protocol for this.

There is a difference between an ancestor who comes through in a dream needing help (or offering you help) and one who is stuck on an old grudge or in a revenge pattern. These ancestors will try to wrest something from you. The previous message of "Help me, I am still suffering" is different than "I am still enraged, and you have to finish the job for me." This type of inheritance may include a history of violence, shunning, scapegoating, or banishment; someone was hurt or hurt others, and they are still upset about it. We know that hurt people hurt people, and it is important to keep that message from being passed down.

This desire for revenge is not yours to carry out, and acting on it may serve to perpetuate the enmity. These are ancestors who died without resolving their anger or grief, and they are in effect "haunting" you with their requests or demands for you to finish their work. Think of the infamous feuds between the Hatfields and McCoys, or families during the Civil War who were divided between the North and the South (some to this day), or unexplained cutoffs in your own family. Shakespeare wrote about this too: The generational feud between the Capulets and the Montagues ultimately led to the deaths of both Romeo and Juliet before their families could resolve their conflict.

The desire for revenge freezes grief. Long-standing personal feuds and strife block the flow of grief and keep people stuck in an endless loop of frozen pain. Unmetabolized grief often transforms into some form of accusatory blame or even violence. When unresolved negative emotions get stuck and are carried beyond the grave, they can morph into rage and revenge for real or imagined wrongs. Your job, then, is not to continue to act out this family saga, but to find a way to recognize and balance the wrongs and hurts so you can send the ancestral spirits back to the light, where they can finally rest and be healed.

One of my favorite book titles is *It Didn't Start with You: How Inherited Family Trauma Shapes Who We Are and How to End the Cycle*. In this book, Mark Wolynn describes this pattern of intergenerational inheritances as both the "family body" and the "family mind."[12] Wolynn cites German psychotherapist Bert Hellinger, the founder of Constellation Work, as evidence that we share a family consciousness with those who came before us.[13] This family consciousness is often so embedded in the unconscious mind that we are unaware of it.

Constellation Work, which is a form of psychodrama, helps people reenact and embody old patterns that need to be healed. Psychodrama enactments allow us to create scenes, like scenes in a play, that depict the issue or dilemma we are struggling with. This work is often done with a group of people, each of whom take a different role in a dream scene; this approach is frequently used in dream circles. Constellation Work allows us to embody every being, every animal, and each object or landscape in a dream and speak as if from their voice. As we enliven these components, it gives us even more perspective and information.

---

12. Wolynn, *It Didn't Start with You*, 25, 40.
13. Wolynn, *It Didn't Start with You*, 44–45.

EXERCISE
Identifying Old Grudges

This exercise will be particularly useful for you if you are experiencing nightmares or upsetting dreams, or if you are aware of cut-offs in your family, especially those that are not fully explained. It is crucial to keep yourself safe and separated when you put your attention on this information.

Before you begin the exercise, if you know of family cut-offs, take some time to ask your living relatives about any grudge-holding ancestors. What was their life like? In particular, does your living relative know what unresolved upset the ancestor may have taken with them to the grave? Then, proceed as follows.

1. Surround yourself with the sapphire-blue container of light, healing, and repair. At first, your job is just to become aware, stay out of the fray, and determine what your ask will be.

2. Next, if you know about this part of your history, attend to who had a fight or argument. With who, and why? Who was shunned, shamed, or scapegoated? Who was unable to forgive? What is the back story here? If you had no living relatives to ask about family cut-offs, tune in to what you do know about your family history, and pay attention to what feels connected or relevant for you to get a general sense that you can still work with. This information can provide a source of understanding as to where this angry figure in your dreams comes from. You can then more easily do grudge-healing work, help them let go, and send them back over the veil to be healed.

3. Once you have answers, keep this information in a safety box in your mind. Better yet, write it down and put it away until you are ready and have the resources to do this healing work. A protocol can be found in chapter 8.

Chapter One

Message Six: "Carry On My Name and Gifts to Your Children and Your Children's Children. Remember."

There is one last message the ancestors may want to convey by appearing in your dreams: to rekindle their light. How can you honor your ancestors' memories, pass on their gifts, and remember them for future generations? If they continue to show up in your dreams or little hints of them keep nudging you in your waking life, it may be a message that your ancestors want to be recalled, remembered, and honored. In Jewish tradition and the Torah, one of the key messages repeated over and over is *m'dor l'dor*, "from generation to generation." This is one of the ways we all survive in the world: by passing on the gifts from our ancestors. Moreover, you can heal the legacy of an ancestor who needs healing before passing their memory down to the next generation. My congregational rabbi, Josh Breindel, says that remembering is a devotional act.

There are many ways you can honor and remember your ancestors, including naming your children after them. You may use the ancestor's full name, the translation of their name in your native tongue, or even the first letter of their name. My friend Shari took her grandmother's name as her own last name at a transitional time in her life. She was finding her own way, separating from some of the challenging legacies of her family of origin, and she had committed to healing from a series of traumatic losses that included the loss of her home, marriage, and health. Shari's Nana Rose was the only family member in whose presence she consistently felt genuine compassion, tenderness, and kindness, so to honor her grandmother, Shari legally changed her last name to Rose. In addition to honoring her grandmother of that name, Shari was choosing to rise, to transcend, to overcome. The name Rose spoke to Shari's desire to elevate her spirit and to help others do so as well. Nana Rose would be proud that this was the purpose of her new namesake, and she periodically shines through in Shari's dreamscapes.

Another way to honor your ancestors is by using artifacts you have inherited from them in your daily life or in moments of celebration. You could cook the foods you learned from them or collect their recipes, in their own handwriting if you are lucky. Every time I make date nut bread or four-bean casserole, I smile as I see my mom's beautiful cursive handwriting on the recipe card. You could plant the same flowers, herbs, or vegetables in your garden that they planted in theirs. Of course, you can honor their memory in many other ways, including music, art, ritual, ceremony, and shrine building. At our core, humans are still hunter-gatherers. This may be why we tend to accumulate tchotchkes, little pieces of the lives of our parents and grandparents that we just can't let go of. These objects contain meaning and memories. When I clean a home after a loved one's death, I often spend much more time than I thought I would, as each throw pillow, dinner plate, and item of clothing brings back memories and stories.

Music is another memory keeper. The music of your ancestors, of your family lineage, is another way to keep connected. By singing and/or playing their music, you connect to the language they spoke and the melodies of their lives and lands, and the music can get under regular layers of consciousness. At a recent song workshop I participated in, we were asked by the instructor to listen with our bodies to a tune, beyond the words, and to get a sense of where the tune took us in time and place. It was very powerful.

Once you have created a means of remembering, honoring, and passing down an ancestor's legacy to your descendants, you will likely get a confirmatory dream or message of some kind. This is the ancestor's way of acknowledging you or thanking you. After my colleague Anna told her daughter about their Cherokee heritage and showed her their family tree, she dreamt of a white feather. Anna knew in her bones that this was her grandfather's acknowledgment that his legacy was being passed on and honored.

Remembering your ancestors may also be about integrating a fuller sense of their lives and stories. As you converse with them, work with them, walk and talk and dream with them, you may learn more about them. For example, you may learn about hidden acts of kindness they performed, the reason and rationale behind their apparent cruelties, and the traumas or griefs they suffered. Learning this information can help account for behaviors that feel difficult or unexplainable.

Chapter One

Inviting Your Ancestors in Through Dream Incubation

Sometimes the ancestors are just waiting to be invited to show up, whether in your dreams or in waking life through synchronicities and symbols. Dream incubation is one way of inviting them in. This is the practice of dreaming with intention, sometimes called "dreaming on purpose."

Dream incubation has been around for millennia. The dream temples of Asclepius in ancient Greece attracted pilgrims from far and wide. Visitors traveled to these temples to heal body, mind, and spirit. They underwent a ritual purification with the temple priests and priestesses, then slept overnight in the temple with their quest for healing as the intention for their dreams to respond to. Small non-venomous snakes were let loose in the night; they were said to whisper the dreams in the visitors' ears. In the morning, temple guides would help visitors interpret their dreams.[14]

Variations on traveling to a sacred site for powerful dreams or visions abound in spiritual literature. The Bible and the Koran are full of these journeying stories, as are the teaching stories of many indigenous groups around the world.

For our purposes, travel and snakes are not necessary—but intention is. With intention, you can point your dreaming self in the direction you want to go. If your goal is to connect with your ancestors, start with that intention and invite them in.

> **EXERCISE**
>
> *Dream Incubation to Connect with Ancestors*
>
> Use this exercise before going to bed if you want to connect with your ancestors. Connecting with ancestors in your dreams can be as simple as writing or speaking a sentence of intention before you go to sleep.
>
> 1. Spend some time thinking about who you would like to invite into your dream. Be clear about who you are inviting, whether it is a specific person or a general request for someone from your lineage. Some souls have finished

---

14. Patton, "Dream Incubation."

their work here in peace and are pleased to be contacted and invited, while others may be hurting or angry. Use this protocol to connect with a benevolent ancestor.

2. Once you have decided who you would like to invite into your dream, surround yourself with protection so that you don't inadvertently invite in overwhelming or malevolent beings or entities. Create your container of light, as discussed earlier in this chapter.

3. Set your intention. You can write it in your dream journal or say it aloud; speak in at least a whisper so your ears can hear what your mouth is saying. If you aren't sure what to say, use the following intention: "As I surround myself with the blue light of protection and clarity, I invite my [mother, father, grandmother, brother, etc.] to visit me tonight. May they come in peace and depart in peace, and may they know that I love them and would welcome a visit."

4. Your ancestor may or may not visit on your first invitation. Don't give up! Keep inviting them. Modify the words in your intention if need be. If an ancestor does make contact, it may be while you are sound asleep or in that liminal space between waking and sleeping. Your ancestor may visit as themselves, or their presence may be a voice, sound, smell, or touch. Don't dismiss any form of contact. You will recognize something specific that is their signature.

A Dream or a Visit?

When dreaming of the departed, many people speak of it as a visit rather than a dream. Visits are reported particularly often in the first weeks after someone dies. What is the difference between a dream and a visit? In a dream, what you see is a character who is part of your dream story. It may be that the dream character is clearly your mother, but she is acting within the dream along with known or unknown dream people. Or there may be a character in the dream who does not look like your dad but, somehow, you know it is him.

By contrast, in a visit, you will likely have a powerful and visceral felt sense of your loved one's presence. You can feel the essence of your beloved right there with you, as if they were still alive. A visit is usually more vivid, more intense, more colorful, and more real. You may hear their voice or feel the touch of their hands as concrete occurrences. Often, there is a numinosity in either the visit or the person, a sense of light, glowing, shining, shimmering, or larger-than-life brightness.

Sometimes a visit comes in other bodies. A bright red cardinal came and tapped at my mom's bedroom window every day for a week after my stepdad Bud died. This had never happened before, and it's never happened since. My mom was convinced that it was her beloved husband. We gladly joined her in this, and whenever a cardinal visits my house, we say, "Hi Bud." It always makes me smile. In many cultures and in folklore, birds are said to carry the spirit of the departed to the living.

Sometimes visitations occur spontaneously; other times, they only come by invitation. My hairdresser reports frequent visits from her departed mom and sister. She is, like me, a thin-boundaried person who easily crosses thresholds. One day, her husband (who works with her in the salon) overheard us talking and piped in, "Mine never visit." I suggested to him that they might just be waiting for an invitation, if he was interested in a visit. He replied that it didn't really matter that much to him. His ambivalence and lack of interest in having them show up was probably part of the reason he hadn't experienced this. We all have different relationships with the dreaming world as well as with relatives.

Dreamer and author Mike Marble shares, "I ask if they have requested a dream with the person they desire to connect with. They often seem surprised by this inquiry. Just as someone waits for an invitation to dinner, some of us don't assume an unannounced visit is warranted. Remembering our dreams and setting an intention to meet up with that person increases the likelihood of it occurring. It's a two-way street so to speak."[15] I love the analogy of waiting for a dinner invitation, rather than just showing up at someone's house. Seems that there might be a protocol that some ancestors prefer to follow!

---

15. Marble, *How to Have a Good Life After You're Dead*.

TWO

BRING HOME MY BONES

"Bring home my bones when you depart from this land"
Bring home too the bones of the Bright Ones
The shining stars of your history
—*Linda Yael Schiller*

The working title I had for this book was *Bring Home My Bones*. It morphed into a chapter title instead, but the theme of the bodies and bones of the ancestors and dreamwork has stuck with me. In the United States, we use the expression "I can feel it in my bones" when we have an aha moment or when we deeply know something. This is a part of the embodied nature of ancestral dreams; there is a "bone-knowing" about them, one that either needs to be embraced, let go of, or healed, depending on the nature of the legacy.

Bones and Marrow

Bones contain the essence of who we are. Bone marrow produces red blood cells that oxygenate the entire body, white blood cells that help fight disease, platelets needed for clotting, and stem cells.

Bone marrow holds the blueprints that contain a person's history and their future. The remnants of your ancestors are contained within this marrow, within the red blood cells that contribute to your physical traits, personality, and quirks. These red blood cells also contain literal traces of past events—both positive and negative—that have altered your family genetics. (We will talk more about this in chapter 3.)

Bones are not only a solid scaffolding of the body, but as stated above, they contain the living, growing tissue that produces marrow. Therefore, the essence of human life is contained in bone and marrow. Bones are the last earthly traces of the dead, and since they seem to last forever, bones symbolize eternal life. Conversely, in the multilayered way of dreamwork, they also may represent mortality and the transitory nature of life.

Stem cells heal. They are the only cells within the body that can create other cell types; they are the body's raw material. Bone marrow and embryonic tissue create many types of specialized cells and offer opportunities for healing forms of cancer and blood disorders. Every type of blood cell starts as a stem cell. Fittingly, when stem cells in a lab reproduce, they are called "daughter cells." How appropriate for our consideration of the intergenerational transmission of blessings or pain from parent to child!

So, veneration of your ancestral bones makes organic sense. Bones contain the essence, the source of who we are. Your bones contain connections between your personal, ancestral, global, and earth-based traumas and gifts. Not only are bones the living artifacts of the ancestors, but many traditions consider bones to be a link between the physical and spiritual self. As the locus of life, bones are said to have mystic powers ranging from healing to divination to birth and rebirth.

Many cultures around the world have some means of honoring the bones of their ancestors, whether through burial, shrine making, bringing good luck, or warding off evil spirits. Some traditions use "throwing the bones" as a means of divination, which also is one of the many functions of a dream. Christian saints may be honored with reliquaries that contain a bone or the bone of a saint. Human bones are often kept as relics for veneration and remembrance. As the last earthly traces of the departed, bones can also symbolize the wholeness of a person, their kinship, or their strength.

You can dream for yourself, for your ancestors, and for the world. Your nightmares may contain the fingerprints of intergenerational traumas. Ancestral connections may be personal, biological, cultural, animal, or rooted in the land. Many of us don't live on the land where our ancestors' bones are buried, so finding a way to connect with them metaphorically or symbolically will be crucial.

In the Bible, bringing the bones of the ancestors back to their homeland was an ubiquitous request. It was the request from Jacob to his son Joseph (the great dreamer), who wanted to be buried with his ancestors. Joseph then repeated this request to his brothers and children and made them swear an oath to do the same. This duty was passed on to Moses, who led the people out of slavery in Egypt during the Exodus back to the land where their ancestors were buried.[16] It was crucial for their literal bones be buried with their forebearers. This is something to consider as you contemplate what bone means to you, both the literal as well as the metaphysical aspects of bone.

Your Bone Memories

Once you have created a means of remembering, honoring, and passing down a legacy to your descendants, you will often get a confirmatory dream or message of some kind as an ancestral acknowledgment or thank you. A workshop I led in October 2023 included a waking dream exercise: I asked participants to take a slow, silent walk outside and to be on the lookout for signs and signals related to the question they were seeking guidance on, also known as a waking dream incubation. I decided to complete the exercise as well.

The waking dream question I incubated was "What can I do to help heal this fractured world of ours from war, as the world explodes in large and small ways across the globe?" As a citizen of the world, all sentient beings are my ancestors, and in the Ukraine and the Middle East, the descendants of my personal ancestors are clearly suffering. In that moment, many places in need of healing were close to my heart and legacy. It was a big question, but even asking it helped me feel less helpless. And, in the context of intergenerational healing, I knew that being of help now was going to help my descendants in the future.

As I walked and looked and listened, I saw one of those Halloween decorations replete with bones right next door to my workshop, proclaiming "Rest in Peace." Not only did I notice the bones and the engraved tombstone, but as I walked a bit further, I chuckled as I caught sight of

---

16. See Genesis 47:30, Genesis 50:25, Exodus 13:19, and Joshua 24:32.

a bumper sticker that read "Coexist," with each letter symbolizing a different religion or ideology. The question I had incubated was broad and vague, so my answer came in kind. Shortly, you will get to practice this in a more focused way.

So, what might it mean to rest in peace and to learn to coexist? And, for that matter, what might it mean to rest in peace while we are still alive? After this waking dream incubation, I found concrete ways to act. First, I donated to agencies who were on the ground in warzones helping with medical care, access to food, and trauma recovery. Then, I contacted a dream podcaster I knew and offered to do an episode on healing trauma and nightmares, particularly when the trauma is ongoing rather than a thing from the past. Post-traumatic stress disorder, which occurs after a traumatic event has passed, is not the same as experiencing ongoing or acute trauma, and I felt it was important to offer some practices that differentiated this. These were two things I could do to help.

When you dream of your ancestors, you are responding to the memories poking through the veil between worlds, reminding or insisting or encouraging you to take some kind of action. When these memories stay buried in your unconscious, you risk not remembering or learning from your past. However, when you acknowledge and honor these calls, you can reap the harvest of your ancestral gifts while also healing trauma. By attending to your dreams and paying attention to synchronicities, you allow your ancestors to emerge in your consciousness. Then, you can be intentional about your work and about sharing their gifts.

The Spiritual Side of Bones

Flesh and bone can symbolize the earth and our connection to the land we live on. Native Hawaiians believed that bones were the primary physical embodiment of a person. After death, the deceased's bones were considered sacred, since the *mana*, or spiritual essence of the person, resided in the bones. Burial of the bones of the deceased was considered a "planting" by traditional Native Hawaiians, as this planting of the bones nourished the soil that crops were later planted in.[17] In this way, the full circle of life was honored: The bones of the ancestors nourished the lives of the descendants, and each cared for and protected the other.

In the late sixteenth century, bones from cemeteries in Evora, Portugal, were relocated and displayed in the Chapel of Bones. Upon visiting the site, my friend Lisa wrote, "Rather than interring the bones that were displaced behind closed doors, the monks, who were concerned about society's values at that time, put them on display embedded in the portals of the doorways and some of the walls, enabling visitors to meditate on the transience of material things in the presence of death."[18] This message was inscribed above the chapel door: *Nos ossos que aqui estamos pelos vossos esperamos*, which roughly translates to "We bones that are here, for yours we wait."[19] I don't think it gets clearer than that.

Mending the ancestral web and establishing (or re-establishing) the relationship between the living and the dead were core principles of Carl Jung's autobiography, *Memories, Dreams, Reflections*, and his seminal work, *The Red Book*. The core of your own belief system, the marrow of your worldview, will show up as you flesh out the dreams and visions of your ancestors. It is important to note that your spiritual ancestors may not have a direct link to your genealogy—that is, they may not be part of your biological family. When you listen at the level of bone-knowing, you may discover spiritual ancestors that have no relation to your family tree. For example, you may connect with your spiritual family and/or the spiritual roots of the land you live on. Watching and listening for the synchronicities between your dream life, your waking life, and your creative process may open you up to worlds of connection and blessings that you didn't realize were gifts from your ancestral guides.

My friend Maya was struck by these kinds of synchronicities. For many years, she had studied therapeutic practices with a teacher named Samuel. He who was a powerful mentor for her. Recently, Maya recognized there were uncanny similarities between her own family history and Samuel's.

---

17. Ayao, "Native Burials."
18. Lisa Korklan, email message to author, November 12, 2023.
19. "Bones Chapel in Evora, Sao Francisco Church."

Both Samuel and Maya's mother had experienced the traumas of persecution, escaped from Nazi Europe in the 1930s, and emigrated to America as young teens. Maya discovered that Samuel and her mother came to America at precisely the same age, thirteen, and settled in the same state. However, the two had very different experiences as they aged. For Maya's mother, the past still existed as a present-day terror. Her parenting was influenced by her unresolved traumas of loss, hiding, running, displacement, and fear. She had not been able to do her own healing—she may not have known that was an option. Maya's mother suffered from PTSD, and she had a felt sense of fear in her daily life.

In contrast, Samuel had been able to help heal his past thanks to his work with the deep unconscious, his dreams, and spiritual pathways. Therefore, he no longer defined or identified himself by his traumas and was able to live in the world in a way that Maya's mother had not been able to. Samuel guided others using his own journey of healing and served as a role model for Maya; the wounded healer is a common motif in archetypical psychology. Maya felt in her bones that Samuel was a spiritual elder who was meant to help her learn and heal from the intergenerational traumas in her own family. Sometimes, if we are lucky, our spiritual elders are still with us and serve as living ancestral role models while we are alive.

Here is another example of the gift of alternative role models in adulthood. Recently, my dear friend John recounted that he found role models for what it meant to be an adult man in his Jungian-based men's group. He had been looking for this kind of role model for quite some time. John's father had been a good dad while the children were young, but parenting them well into adulthood was beyond his capacity: John's father had suffered a head injury while in the service, and although he recovered, there were still gaps and missing pieces in his cognitions and behaviors. He died when John was in his forties and had just started parenting his own child. I was so pleased to hear that John was given a second chance to connect with adult male role models as "living ancestors."

Full Circle: Borscht and Bones

As you begin to work with your dreams, you will be able to find more and more layers of meaning. No matter how strong of a dreamer you are, you could always benefit from at least one other companion plumbing the depths of your dreams. Strong dreamwork is often about the power of broad association, which is why dream-working with others adds depth and perspective.

For example, in the introduction, I shared the following dream:

I am learning the borscht recipe from a chef. It seems that we needed a piece of equipment called a shredder to make the soup. The chef helps me locate one. After that, I am in charge of teaching my students how to do it. They aren't getting it right, so we have to start over from scratch now that we have the shredder.

When I unpacked this dream with my friend Diana, I discovered it had many more layers than I initially realized. Using the free associative nature of dreamwork, one association lead to another.

As I focused my attention on my dream, I first associated it with my friend Geneva, who had given me a recipe for a delicious borscht soup. Her name reminded me of the word *generative*, of generations, and the Roman goddess of wisdom, Minerva.

Another layer of this dream had to do with the fact that the bones of some of my ancestors are still in the Ukraine. In my dream, I was connecting with the bones of my ancestors, with my roots. And in certain parts of the world, beets are called *beetroots*.

A chef was teaching me how to make the food of my ancestors. We needed a particular tool to do it right: a shredder. As I reflected, I asked myself, *What is a shredder?* Instinctively, I answered that a shredder is a tool that transforms something that is hard or inedible into something that is edible and nutritious. It makes the food placed within it accessible. Connecting with the legacy of my ancestors nourishes me. Additionally, a shredder mixes ingredients together to blend them into something greater, the sum of all parts.

And, on another layer, a shredder shreds. It causes pain. It tears things apart. When people are hurt on a heart level, they might say, "I feel shredded." My ancestors—and likely yours—must have felt shredded at times. So many of us have family legacies that include pain.

At the end of the dream, I was teaching my students how to use the shredder to make borscht. I was passing this recipe's legacy on to the next generation, helping them remember by literally ingesting the rooted food of the past. Remembering is reconnecting, and it puts the pieces back together.

Finally, to connect this dream to present-day life, I was recently contacted by Jose, a member of the IASD dream organization. Jose worked as an American aid volunteer in the Ukraine, and he told me that he was using my books to help the survivors of the war heal from their nightmares and trauma. Full circle. I got to pay it forward and bring some small measure of healing to a country that once persecuted my ancestors, hopefully offering healing to my past, the present, and the future survivors of this war.

* * *

Each culture has ancestral stories of their own, often connected with the bones of their ancestors in some way. What makes bones and lands and dream themes sacred for a person? You may have lived in an area for a long time. The bones of your ancestors could be buried in a certain land. You may feel deep, unexplainable spiritual roots to a certain location, perhaps from another lifetime. So many things can contribute to the sense of the numinous in personal and familial legacies.

EXERCISE
Bone-Knowing

Use the following exercise when you are interested in connecting with your ancestors through a guided waking meditation. Set an intention to receive whatever messages you need to hear from your ancestors.

1. Close your eyes. Sit and breathe quietly.

2. When you feel ready, begin a body scan, starting with the top of your head (or, if you prefer, you can start with your feet and work up). In your mind's eye, focus your attention on slowly scanning over your body, resting for a moment on each part. Feel a gentle felt sense, a noticing, as you put your attention on the crown of your head,

face, neck and throat, shoulders, down your arms to each finger and thumb, then up to your chest and upper back, stomach and lower back, hips and pelvis, thighs, knees, legs, tops of the feet, toes, and soles of the feet. Notice how your skin and organs are supported by your skeleton, by your bones.

3. Next, tune in to the innermost part of your bones: the marrow, the essence of your life (and the lives of your ancestors and descendants). Notice this source of ultimate creativity and connection.

4. In this trancelike, waking-dream state, revisit your intention to connect with your ancestors. Receive these messages from this place of bone-knowing. Take your time, and do not discount anything. Messages may come through in words, images, emotions, or sensations in your body; a message might be a quick blip or a long narrative. Learn what you need to learn in a way that serves your highest purpose. Bookmark the learnings so you can return to them during nighttime dream incubation.

5. When you are ready, come back fully into the present. Stretch or shake it out, drink some water, and write down your experience. Later tonight, use this information as your blueprint for incubating dreams to further your knowledge and guide you to the actions you need to take to heal your family line. Repeat this for as many nights as you need to.

THREE

EPIGENETICS AND HEALING THE DREAMS WE CARRY FROM OTHERS

> If we understand who and where we came from, genetic destinies can be altered, hopefully for the better.
> —*Jamie Ford,* The Many Daughters of Afong Moy

The relatively new science of epigenetics informs us that events from generations past can still affect us for generations to come. Epigenetics is the study of how behaviors and environments can cause changes that affect our genes. Epigenetic inheritance occurs when we pass on the modulations of our genes. Gene function can change in response to environmental cues and stresses. In this way, stress and struggle can be passed along to future generations, but it is important to remember that so can blessings, gifts, and resilience. You could inherit a tendency to be fragile and vulnerable, or a tendency to be antifragile, strong in the face of the storm. The term *antifragile* was coined by Nassim Nicholas Taleb. Antifragile people and organizations aren't just resilient in times of crisis; they can even become more robust when exposed to stressors, uncertainty, or risk. That is, they can thrive during challenges and in times of uncertainty.

Epigenetic inheritance is malleable and open to change. Unlike genetic changes, epigenetic changes are reversible because they do not irreversibly change your DNA. However, epigenetic changes *can* impact how your body reads a DNA sequence.

Chapter Three

We Can "Reverse the Curse"

The knowledge that epigenetic changes are reversible means, in short, we can heal. That is key for this work. Healing the effects of current and past trauma in your lifetime can prevent that trauma from trickling down to subsequent generations. You can embody the phrase "the buck stops here" as you work with your dreams, memories, emotions, and body.

Epigenetics offers hope that you can still get closure on long-passed events. Vamik Volkan is an international psychoanalyst who studies the effects of war, terror, and displacement worldwide. He uses the phrase *image deposits* to describe the internalized images of traumatic experiences that can be passed on to subsequent generations.[20] These image deposits can become a part of someone's story even if they themselves did not experience the original trauma. This passing on is an unconscious process. Since dreams are replete with subconscious images and allow you access to the hidden parts of yourself in a way that little else does, dreamwork seems to be a good way to unearth these buried deposits, heal them, and return them, transformed, to the ancestors. Then, replace them in your own life with more affirming ones.

One way we can avoid passing on traumatic experiences is by bringing light to what is transmitted through transgenerational epigenetic inheritance. What is transmitted that was never spoken of, never verbalized, never made conscious? When traumatic events and memories remain unspoken and unacknowledged, they become buried in "crypts" inside of us.[21] In particular, many of us harbor ancestral secrets that were unmentionable, such as premature death, massacre, or violence in some form. Recognizing and naming the secrets of others releases them from the crypt, and the carrier then becomes free to choose their own path.

Another way of looking at this is that past traumas that have not been metabolized by survivors get passed on to subsequent generations. It may require a lot of time and distance for someone to be able to name—and, thus, metabolize and heal—the past. It may take until the third or fourth generation of descendants to release these secrets.

---

20. See Volkan, *A Nazi Legacy*.
21. Schützenberger, *The Ancestor Syndrome*, 46, 141.

A Brief Look at the Science of Epigenetics

During the epigenetic process, tiny chemical tags called methylation are added to or removed from DNA strands in response to life circumstances and the environment in which we are living. Trauma and stressful environments can also create irregularities at another genome level, that of the RNA, which further impacts how genes are expressed in future generations.[22]

The prefix *epi-* means "over" or "upon," so the word *epigenetics* means "over the genes."[23] To clarify this concept, think of the word *epidermis*, the outer layer of skin, which could be understood as "over the dermis"; the dermis is a deeper layer of skin.

Family Legacies

A family is not a singularity; it is a collection of stories and experiences connected to each other. Death doesn't end the connection. Rather, it simply shifts it to a more multidimensional space. After all, time is a spiral winding in and around us. The experiences of your ancestors cling to you, "holding fast to [your] genetic scaffolding."[24] Think of the last time you visited the beach or a sandy area. Even after showering well, it is not unusual to continue to find tiny bits of sand between your toes or in your hair. It is still clinging to the scaffolding of your body. Even if you can't see it, you can feel it. And the more sensitive you are, the more you can feel these sand particles between your toes. It is the same with the overlaps of epigenetic mapping.

In chapter 2, I examined the idea of bone as the scaffolding that contains the stem cells of inheritance. Now, the same concept shows up in epigenetics. It leads to questions such as:

- What aspects of yours are yours alone?
- What is a memory trace, and what might you be carrying around that is not really yours to carry?

---

22. Wolynn, *It Didn't Start with You*.
23. *Merriam-Webster Dictionary*, "epi-," accessed April 29, 2025, https://www.merriam-webster.com/dictionary/epi-.
24. Firestone, *Wounds into Wisdom*, 49.

- When and how can you transform, release, or put down the burdens that you inherited from your ancestors?

Your cellular environment was already present in the egg cells of your mother and grandmother. Little bits of yourself were already present in the ovaries of your grandmother! Women are born with all the egg cells that they will have in life, so that means when your grandmother was pregnant with your mother, the egg cell that would become you was also inside of your grandmother's womb. These cells were then imprinted by the events that your parents and grandparents experienced, with the potential to affect subsequent generations.[25] Three generations literally shared the same biological environment. That affects how genes are expressed and may affect the function of the gene itself. These generational ghosts can show up in your dreams and nightmares, demanding their due.

Epigenetic traces are echoes of the past. As Ford writes, "We're not individual flowers, annuals that bloom and then die. We're perennials. A part of us comes back each new season, carrying a bit of the genus of the previous floret."[26]

Epigenetic Dream Hints and Repeats

It is not simply a figure of speech to say that we feel "haunted" by some dreams or nightmares. There are gaps within us that were left by others' secrets. As mentioned earlier, unspoken events become buried inside us. Many of us carry these events inside of ourselves like a crypt, burying secrets, shame, and pain that could not be spoken.

Many scholars and clinicians underscore that healing intergenerational family trauma begins with awareness. As you tune in, listen to your dreams, and become aware of your patterns, you will begin to increase your awareness. Bearing witness will put you on the path to lasting change, as will practicing healing modalities solo and in the company of others.

The patterns in your life and in your dreams can be connected to your inherited past. You may be recycling both the gifts and the trauma. One way to tune in to potential inherited patterns is by looking at repetitions

---

25. Wolynn, *It Didn't Start with You*, 26.
26. Ford, *The Many Daughters of Afong Moy*, 247.

Epigenetics and Healing the Dreams We Carry from Others

in your dreams. What reoccurs over and over again? You might have the same dream periodically, or there might be certain elements of a dream that repeat.

Do your dreams have recurring images, landscapes, colors, words, characters, or ages? Do you have what are known as *time markers* in your dreams, cues that the dream is set in an earlier part of your life? This may be directly or indirectly communicated by the setting (for example, your elementary school or the house you lived in during childhood), the words (the name of the street you grew up on), or the characters (a friend you have not spoken to in decades). I grew up on Sunrise Street, so a repeating theme for me might be to dream of my street, a sign with the word *Sunrise* on it, a literal sunrise, or a pun on the word, like "son" and an image of something rising, such as bread.

Additionally, do you dream of bodily harm or discomfort over and over? Does a particular relative or friend show up time and time again? Do you find yourself in a particular country, landscape, or time period? If you are dreaming of a particular place, have you ever lived there, or has anyone in your family lived there in the past? If the answer is no and you cannot trace any known connections to the country or people that you dream about over and over, perhaps you are channeling connections from another lifetime, a lifetime that you are not ancestrally connected to in this one.

EXERCISE
Catching the Repeats

If you are unsure whether your dreams have repetitive themes, landscapes, or characters, try this technique. If you are confident that you recognize repeating themes in your dreams, I still recommend completing this exercise for more clarity and a sense of what is calling to you.

This exercise requires you to reference your dream journal. Ideally, this exercise would be done when you have several months, if not years, of dreams to reflect on. However, if you have only been writing down your dreams for a week or two, it's fine to start with that.

1. Gather your dream journal and a few colored pens or markers. Pick a starting point that makes sense to you and begin to skim through what you wrote. When you notice the first repetition—be it of character, place, emotion, storyline, color, or object—highlight that theme in a specific color. As you continue to read, highlight that theme in the same color whenever you encounter it. For example, if you noticed that you frequently dream of your childhood home, each time you encounter that in your writing, you could underline it in blue. If you often had the sense of being lost or chased in a dream, you could underline that in a different color such as red or green.

2. Once you have reached an appropriate ending point, set your markers aside and go back to the page you began on. As you flip through the pages, count the highlighted passages that correspond. Pay attention to what was identical as well as what morphed and changed depending on the dreamscape. Themes will begin to emerge. For example, if you frequently dreamt of your childhood home, who else was there with you? What were you doing? Was it always the same, or did it vary? How so?

3. Then, revisit the highlighted passages once more and really pay attention to the emotional narrative of these repetitive themes, especially for dreams that have to do with your ancestors in some way. The emotional storyline will point you in the direction of your ancestors' need or connection. Do they want to share a warm, loving blessing or advice, or is their message a scary, emotional story of anxiety or fear? Are their messages shouts or whispers?

4. Set aside your dream journal and spend some time meditating on these repeating dreams or themes. Set an inten-

tion. Point yourself in the direction of safety, then knowledge and connection. Open yourself to the messages of your ancestors, especially the ones who have been repeat visitors. Ask yourself the following question: *What am I supposed to learn or know or do for my highest good?*

Silence Keeps Us Stuck on Replay

One of the primary means of healing is speaking up, speaking out, and sharing your pain with others who have been through similar experiences. Trauma breaks connections with others, and healing is about repairing connection. Hence, support groups, organizations, and therapeutic modalities of all kinds have been established in the last half of the century to provide forums for Vietnam veterans, Holocaust survivors, domestic violence survivors, etc. When the trauma and pain of the past remain a secret, the unspoken words and events take on more power than if they were spoken aloud. So many trauma survivors are either unable to put language to their pain or choose not to in the mistaken belief that it is "out of sight, out of mind."

The coping strategy of walling off or sealing over pain is a common human response. Burying the past may seem like a good idea, especially if you are hoping to protect yourself or your children, but this actually has the opposite effect. What is unspoken becomes more powerful and takes on a life of its own. Neurobiologist Daniel Siegel coined the phrase "name it to tame it." This little mantra has helped thousands of survivors begin to heal.

Awareness gives you the opportunity to heal, to reframe, to leave the past in the past, and to learn from it so it does not repeat in the future. There are many ways to learn to speak the unspoken. Attending to your dream life is one means by which you can hear and see what was buried. Bring it to light to be addressed and healed.

The Bequeathment of Legacy Burdens

Victimized or oppressed people parent their children using their lived experiences, and their children—who have less-developed nervous systems—take in this parenting style as truth. Adults may be better able to override these messages. If these messages were not overridden, they passed from generation to generation as a soul wound, buried deep in the psyche. If traumatic experiences get passed down over and over without healing or transformation, they become a familial style or norm. Think of it like this: The original trauma was a rock thrown into a pond, the subsequent generation was affected by the ripples in the water, and the subsequent generations still feel the waves that hit the shoreline. Trauma can be a part of the emotional and energetic landscape of your family system. This is called a *legacy burden* in Internal Family Systems therapy.

For example, your grandparents may have been subject to violence or poverty in their lifetime. Even if they were able to escape dangerous situations, it is likely that traces of these traumas still impacted the way they parented. If the dominant theme of your grandparents' life was safety, the need to constantly be on the lookout was already established. Therefore, your grandparents would have taught their children that same message: The world was not safe, and they needed to constantly be on the lookout, no matter what. Then, your parents would likely have passed that same message on to you. These kinds of messages are carried unconsciously. This is a key component: When a person is unaware, they pass on messages whether they mean to or not.

Attending to the Language of Your Dreams

If English is not the only language you know, pay attention to what language you dream in. There may be moments or periods of time where the language of your ancestors shows up unexpectedly. Perhaps just a few words are embedded in a dream, or maybe the whole dream is in a different language than the one you speak daily. Did you grow up with this language in your household? Do you speak it fluently or only know a few words? Perhaps your parents or grandparents used it as their secret language when they didn't want you to understand what they were talking about; this is not uncommon. It may have been the language of trauma and pain for them, a language that they did not want to pass on to their children. Look at the role of language in your family for clues about its role in your dreamwork.

Epigenetic Dreaming

As I have shared in this chapter, traumatic experiences and responses to trauma can be passed down intergenerationally. Here is one example of how this could show up in dreamwork.

My client, Patty, had a maternal grandmother named Bea. Bea was molested by a male relative during childhood. When Grandma Bea had children of her own, she passed on the messages that men were never to be trusted, that being beautiful was a curse and put people at risk, and that sex was simply a chore to be endured—but only after they were married. Patty's mother grew up hearing these messages and ultimately married at age twenty-two in a sort of arranged marriage.

When Patty herself reached adolescence, her mom passed on coded messages that dating was dangerous. Patty was taught this directly and indirectly, as her mother said things like "Are you really going out wearing that? You won't be safe!" and "You're too pretty. Cover yourself up" and "You know, boys can't be trusted. They only have one thing on their mind."

When Patty came to therapy in her late twenties, her goals were to work on her felt sense of shame about her body, an overeating disorder that began when she was a young teen, and fears of dating and sex. Patty had struggles very similar to those experienced by sexual abuse survivors, but she did not recall any history of sexual assault. Since adolescence, Patty periodically had frightening dreams of being trapped by a shadowy man who groped her under the stairs, but she did not know what those dreams were about or connected to. All Patty knew was that the dreams felt ominous. They were part of what brought her to therapy.

When we created a genogram together, one of the questions I asked Patty was if she knew of any family members who had similar body issues or anxieties. Patty volunteered that her mother certainly did, but that she didn't know where they might have originated. After constructing a genogram, Pat felt empowered to talk to her mother with the genogram in hand as a prop.

As they talked, Patty's mom revealed what her own mother—Patty's Grandma Bea—had once told her long ago: Grandma Bea's uncle trapped her under the stairs and groped her on several occasions. The secret was finally out.

Chapter Three

Grandma Bea's actual circumstances were eerily similar to Patty's dreams. Epigenetic layers can show up in dreams and through the collective unconscious, a term coined by Carl Jung that speaks to knowledge and information passed down through nonlinear and uncanny ways of knowing. This pattern had persisted through three generations of women in Patty's family. With the confirmation that her fears and nightmares did not originate in her own life, Patty was able to recognize that these fears were a result of her mother's and grandmother's experiences, messages, and parenting styles.

With time, Patty was able to let go of the beliefs and behaviors that were not actually hers to carry. She went on to have a satisfying dating life and married someone she loved, and she knows that she will be teaching her own daughters a different message when they get older. Patty stopped this pattern from being passed on. Moreover, Patty's story is a good reminder to not make assumptions about your dreams or life patterns, but to continue to investigate what they mean until you feel a sense of truth and rightness.

Some dream themes that are traumatic can be transformed through humor. Something that is key in understanding dreams is their emotional narrative, the emotional story that accompanies the events. In the following example, the dream felt amusing, not frightening.

My client Meagan's grandparents survived the great Irish potato famine. To this day, Meagan and her mom are extremely careful never to waste food and to save all leftovers. Sometimes, Meagan dreams of little potato eyes winking at her. Meagan quickly made the connection between her dreams and the potato famine. They were, after all, both about potatoes. This kind of dream is also called a *confirmatory dream*, as it confirms something that we believe is true.

When we unpacked this dream message, she decided that the potato eyes were winking at her to let her know that she and her family did in fact survive, and the humorous wink was a green light to go forward in life without fear of starvation.

Repetitive Intergenerational Trauma

In English, we have the term *old soul*, for better or for worse. You may know a person whose soul seems to carry old knowledge or old pain. Perhaps they have knowledge seemingly beyond their years, or there is a layer of pain or grief beyond their known life experiences.

Studies have shown that many second- and third-generation Holocaust survivors exhibit the same types of intrusive and violent nightmares that their parents or grandparents experienced, even though they themselves did not endure the concentration camps.[27] Even if you and your parents did not experience violence, starvation, or loss, the traces of those memories remain in your energetic field through the epigenetic shifts in your DNA.

Patterns may also be passed on through the repetition of reactions and responses, especially if those reactions or responses were useful coping strategies when the original traumas occurred. With that being said, the path of an inherited trauma can be random: "You never know who will get it, but someone will."[28] Some people are more affected than others, even amongst those who grew up in the same household. Sometimes, family trauma skips a generation altogether and sinks its teeth into the next generation. It seems that this is more common when there has been silence, when the stories were not told nor the losses grieved.

Both Meagan's and Patty's stories are examples of patterns being passed on by family members. Parenting styles—such as being suspicious of men or never wasting a morsel of food—developed after being parented by the children of trauma survivors. Thus, the subsequent generation passed on both direct and indirect messages related to this trauma. These messages then became a learned response. It is common for these messages to show up in dreams and nightmares, even if you yourself did not experience the original traumatic event that started this chain of reactions.

Patterns can get passed on in waking life as well. My stepfather, Bud, lost his father when he was only nineteen years old. It was the late 1940s, and Bud's mother was overwhelmed and grieving. As a result, she instructed

---

27. Yehuda and Lehrner, "Intergenerational Transmission of Trauma Effects"; Yehuda et al., "Holocaust Exposure Induced Intergenerational Effects on FKBP5 Methylation."
28. Shafak, *The Forty Rules of Love*, 128.

her children to be uber-independent. Bud married young, and when he was still shy of thirty, he suddenly lost his wife to an aneurysm. Their three children were ten, seven, and six years old.

With the help of his own mother, Bud raised his children to be very independent and dissuaded them from talking about their feelings, much like how he was raised. Bud was a marvelous father in many ways, but he minimized the effect losing their mother had on his children. Of course, Bud struggled with the loss of his wife, but he also had a history of unresolved grief. Statements such as "You can do it," "You're fine," and "We don't need to talk about this with anyone" were the messages Bud got and gave. That uber-independence was a good thing—until it wasn't.

Bud's daughter struggled with depression as a teen, but no one really noticed. She went to school and functioned, but when she came home from school, she slept all afternoon until dinner. It wasn't until years later that she recognized it for what it was. When she was in a difficult marriage, she didn't get help or support from Bud until the very end; his mindset was that she had to figure it out herself, like he had to as a young man. Eventually, after attending therapy, Bud's daughter was able to recognize this family pattern and did not ignore warning signs of her own children's mental health issues—she got them the help they needed right away.

Trauma dysregulates the ability to cope and function optimally in life. A trauma response may cause you to react to a historical event as if it was happening right now. The past and the present become entangled and confused, much as they do in a dream state. Dreamtime and trauma time are remarkably similar.

My client Marina, who is an author, was recently asked to appear on television to promote her book. Her knee-jerk response to that invitation was panic that went way beyond typical performance anxiety. The next night she had the following dream:

> As I make my way to the television studio for my interview, I know that I will be killed if I go through with it. The only recourse is to run home immediately and cancel the show.

As we unpacked Marina's dream and her reaction, she traced it back to generations of family history. Marina frequently got the message "Don't be visible, it isn't safe. The only safety is in hiding who you are." While processing this dream, Marina was able to remember numerous messages about assimilation, "passing," and not standing out, all of which she received from her parents and grandparents.

Marina shared that her family had fled pogroms in Eastern Europe at the turn of the previous century. While this was not Marina's current reality, it registered as such in her unconscious until we could identify the sources. Once identified, Marina could then use active dreamwork to "upgrade the operating system" of her unconscious and dreaming mind. She began to identify what was in the past and what was in the present, what belonged in her own life and what belonged in generations past. I will teach you how to do this in chapter 7.

Epigenetics are patterns. So are family legacy burdens. Not repeating old patterns is the equivalent of tracing new neural pathways in the brain, pathways that become deeper and stronger than the previous ones. Old patterns have taken up so much time and energy not only in your life, but in the lives of your parents, grandparents, and others. The associated neural pathways are already well-established, so you will need to keep practicing so you do not fall back into old patterns. To truly change a pattern, you will need to institute a new one. Replace the old patterns of trauma and loss with something else that is new and generative. And if repetition enhances the neural pathways of trauma, we can also use repetition to enhance life-affirming, healing patterns.

From the point of view of epigenetics, inherited patterns can either be turned on or off. Thus, epigenetics could activate overwhelming anxiety or sufficient coping skills in the same person at different times, according to the external or internal environmental factors. As emphasized by Yehuda and Bierer, "Integrating epigenetics into a model that permits prior experience to have a central role in determining individual differences is also consistent with a developmental perspective of PTSD vulnerability."[29] In other words, you will be less vulnerable to developing PTSD in the face of stress when you are free from unhealthy inherited patterns.

---

29. Yehuda and Bierer, "The Relevance of Epigenetics to PTSD," 432.

Finally, the study and knowledge of epigenetics opens a more optimistic view of health and disease in offspring of trauma survivors. Since the science of epigenetics conveys that human beings are not predestined to suffer, but are highly malleable creatures, they are able to reverse the deleterious effects of trauma and find some closure to the endless multi-generational saga.

These transformations may be achieved through a variety of sleeping and waking dreamwork methods, through therapeutic interventions, through new supplements or medications, or a combination of them all. Instead of succumbing to the emotional effects of the past tragedies, we can search and find some kind of personal transformation journey that gives new meaning to our legacy, realizing that not only is it up to us to find ways to heal old patterns, but that it is possible.

> **EXERCISE**
> *Letting Go of the Rocks*
> This exercise should be done with someone who can help facilitate the physical aspects, hold the space, and bear witness to your experience. You could choose a friend, a family member, or a mental health professional you are working with. This exercise could also be done in a group setting; members can take turns offering the rocks.
>
> Before you begin, gather a pile of small- or medium-sized rocks that you can hold in your arms. If rocks are not available, a stack of books or even small pots and pans will do—anything that has some weight, but that can still be held in your arms.
>
> 1. Stand, or sit comfortably if standing is not possible. Take a few deep breaths.
> 2. Name the legacy burdens that you are carrying. Are there family cut-offs, past traumas, hurts or neglect, a history of persecution, or emotions you have that are connected to long-ago events? Speak them aloud.
> 3. When you have finished, have your partner say something like, "These events and feelings belong to genera-

Epigenetics and Healing the Dreams We Carry from Others

tions past. They do not belong to the present time, but you are still carrying them." Your partner should then ask, "Are you ready to feel literally what you have been carrying emotionally?"

4. Once you are ready, cradle your arms against your abdomen. Your partner should start to pile rocks in your arms. Have your partner do this slowly so you don't get overwhelmed or injured. Each time your partner adds another rock, they should ask you, "Can you hold any more? Should we stop here?" Keep doing this until you say "Stop" or until you run out of rocks.

5. When you have reached your capacity, take a moment and notice what it is like to hold all these rocks, all these "issues." What does it feel like? For example, you might feel annoyed, or sad, or constricted, or heavy. Name all the sensations and emotions that come to mind.

6. Then, let your arms drop and release all the rocks. If you are not ready to do that, notice why not: Why do you want to hold on to all, or some, of these rocks/issues/emotions that you have already named as not yours? If you feel guilty for letting them go, then you've earned another rock on the pile for guilt!

7. Once you have dropped all (or some) of the rocks, notice how your body feels. Notice how much lighter you feel.

8. Gently set down any rocks that you were not yet ready to let go of. Shake yourself out. Move your arms and legs about. Then, ask yourself, *How many learnings have I received here?* Let a number instinctively come into your head.

9. Once you have a number, be it one or five or eight, write your learnings down. (If a very large number comes to mind and you can't gather all your learnings right now, write down what you can, and commit to writing down

the rest later in the day.) This is what you now know to be true, having let go of those burdens.

10. If your learnings don't already contain an action step, go back and add at least one concrete thing you will do now that you have been freed of this family legacy burden. Action could be a symbolic gesture, a conversation with someone, a piece of art or writing, or volunteer work. The important thing is that the next step involves some kind of action and is meaningful to you.

Our Wise and Wonderful Ones

In addition to inheriting family traumas and pain, you can also inherit the strengths and gifts of your ancestors. If you have pain and suffering as part of your legacy, then you also have a history of gifts, strengths, and wisdom that were passed down as your legacy. We see what we pay attention to, so don't forget to pay attention to your gifts and thank your ancestors for those. Are you good at sports like Uncle Jack? Are you a creative thinker who is ahead of your time like Nona Maria? Do you yearn to adventure and explore like your dad? Are you kind and warm and full of hugs like your mom? These, too, are family legacies.

Alberto Ríos has a beautiful poem that reinforces how powerful legacy is. The gist of his poem "A House Called Tomorrow" is that we carry all of our ancestors inside of us. For every family member who suffered, was troubled, or was troubling, there are many more who were not. It's worth reading the whole thing.[30]

EXERCISE
Gratitude Practice

In the coming chapters, we will examine how to address, honor, and heal all kinds of ancestral messages, but for now, take a moment to thank your wise elders.

---

30. See Ríos, "A House Called Tomorrow."

Epigenetics and Healing the Dreams We Carry from Others

1. Close your eyes. Sit with your feet on the floor, connected to the earth, and your head held erect, connected to the heavens. Quiet your mind and take a few deep breaths.

2. Direct your inner sight to the vision of an ancestor who is wise, who has gifted you in some way, or who you feel blessed by. See them in your mind's eye if you can. (If not, no worries; you can still do this with your felt sense.)

3. From your heart, send this ancestor a message of gratefulness or appreciation. As you do so, notice their response. It may be subtle or strong. It could be a shiver of warmth through your body, the sound of their voice, or their eyes shining as they acknowledge you and the gift of gratitude you have shared with them.

4. Bask in this connection for a while. If you'd like, invite your ancestor to visit your dreams tonight, either to continue the dialogue, to ask for a blessing or advice, or simply to enjoy their company once again.

5. When you feel ready, take a deep breath, open your eyes, and go about your day.

FOUR

RESPECTING DREAMWORK AND ANCESTRY WORLDWIDE, AND THE UNIQUE WORK OF ANCESTRY WITH ADOPTION

> Myths are public dreams, dreams are private myths.
> —*Joseph Campbell*

Honoring dreams and ancestors is part and parcel of many cultures, texts, and spiritual traditions throughout the world, from ancient through modern times. As Joseph Campbell notes, myths and dreams are two halves of a whole. When a person is cut off from their waking visions or sleeping dreams, they are cut off from a part of themself, from a powerful source of information, and from a potential source of connection with their ancestors. The word *oneiromancy* is divination through dreamwork, and this type of prescient dreaming shows up as a powerful means of peering through the ages and across cultures.

In the last few decades, there has been a resurgence of honoring ancient knowledge and practices. While acknowledging that many cultural traditions have been exploited or misappropriated over time, we can learn something from other traditions and their relationships to the dream world by embodying the spirit of curiosity and respect. Doing so will enhance knowledge and a sense of connectedness as beings sharing this world.

For people to heal cultural as well as generational wounds, we need to be more cognizant of how these wounds show up in other traditions. In addition, learning more about traditions and how they are similar or different from each other aids in multicultural awareness, understanding, and healing. Who and where you are from is an integral part of who you are today. Since the beginning of recorded time, most spiritual belief systems have written and/or spoken of legacies and ancestors that the members of the tradition were encouraged to honor, to learn from, to be aware of, to appease, and to remember. When you access your own inherited wisdom and learn some of other peoples', it helps you realize that you are not alone and that the ones who came before you are still with you. Plus, it is fascinating to find the similarities between traditions across the wide expanses of time and space.

It is important to learn about dreamwork in other cultures especially if you have ties to that culture or it has become part of your extended family through marriage, adoption, or ceremony. When a person begins to explore their ancestral past, surprises may show up. Background research or a genetic test may reveal ethnic or racial groups that were or became a family secret. We will see this shortly in the story of my colleague Mia, who first discovered her Native American heritage through her dreams.

In addition, for those who are adopted, have adopted children, or have family members who were adopted, access to biological ancestors may not be available. Therefore, I will also talk about how to research ancestral history when there has been an adoption and how to weave threads of a biological connection—including those of other cultures, as is the case with multiracial adoption—with the traditions of the adoptive family. Adoptive family bonds and history are just as strong and real as biological ones.

The Centrality of Strong Dreamers

Historically, many leaders of various groups, extended families, and spiritual practices were chosen because they were gifted at dreaming and connecting with ancestors. It is a high honor to be considered a good dreamer, and in fact, that is part of the criterion for choosing many shamanic, indigenous, and Earth-based leaders. Thus, dreaming is not simply a nighttime oneiric experience. It is a guidepost for life choices, and it can be approached as an ongoing path toward learning, an awareness of all life, and the active application of knowledge via interactions with others.

To their credit, people are beginning to reclaim this knowledge. Reverence for ancestors and trust in the power of dreaming exist in the world today.

As you read this chapter, be a respectful outsider when learning about traditions that are not your own; enter with curiosity and a non-judgmental approach. Note what you already know about with your own ancestral heritage, traditions, and dreamwork, and consider whether or not you currently have a dreamwork practice. There is a section at the end of the chapter that can help you dive more deeply into your own history and traditions.

Honoring the Wisdom from Hawaiian Culture

Native Hawaiians tuned in to the natural phenomena of the world and attentively noticed patterns. The early Polynesians who followed the stars in their double-hulled canoes to settle in Hawaii came from a long line of voyaging experts and canoe makers. They settled in the Hawaiian Islands around 1100 CE. As close observers of natural phenomena including migratory birds, whales, ocean currents, rainbows, the stars, and the sky, they managed to cross over two thousand miles of ocean in their canoes.[31]

This amazing journey feels like a waking dream state to me. Paying close attention to nature helps connect people to a collective unconscious that can guide and inform us today. This is one of the essential elements of dreamwork: Closely noticing the patterns that show up in your dreams helps you discern their messages.

Moe'uhane is the Hawaiian word for dream and means "soul sleep." The concept of dreams connecting a person to their soul shows up in many cultures, and it is seemingly a part of the collective unconscious. Some elders have shared that they communicate with their ancestral guardians while sleeping, and the most direct way to communicate between the living and the dead is sustained through dreaming. Dreams are therefore seen as one of the best ways to connect with ancestors.

A few years ago, I visited Hawaii and stayed in an Airbnb. As I talked to my host, he confirmed these orientations to nature, dreaming, and the importance of ancestors in his own life. He even came to my *PTSDreams* book reading on Maui and brought his wife and daughter.

---

31. "Early Hawaiians."

My friend Kim, who lived on Maui, confirmed that in her interactions with Native Hawaiians, she learned that ancestor reverence and dream guidance were an integral part of their culture, and these practices were most often done in community. A community of strong dreamers can help hold together the fabric of life and maintain connection in the face of difficulty or even disaster, such as the wildfire disaster of August 2023. Work is still ongoing to heal the land and the people.

African Ancestors and Dreaming

Dreamwork is an essential part of healing in African philosophy and spirituality, as are embodied practices that include ritual, music, and dance. There is a deep and rich story-telling tradition in African countries, part of an ancient oral tradition that includes the telling of dreams to others. An ongoing relationship with the ancestors is a core part of most traditions as well. With that being said, African dreamwork is not monolithic. It is a large continent, and there is continuity of traditions in other lands, so there are many variations. One commonality, though, is the veneration of elders, the future ancestors. Elders are honored and viewed as wisdom keepers.

The West African approach of *ayanmo* is much like the Western conceptualization of the unconscious, thus connecting it with dreamwork. Ayanmo is associated with fate, destiny, and family dynamics, which all find their expression in dreams and dreamwork.[32] The elders help others understand their dreams, and dreams are an expression of personal, ancestral, and spiritual forces operating together through life and the body.

Ritual helps people sustain a relationship with their community, ancestors, the spirits of nature, and the gods. Ritual and ceremony give form to thought and intention. Chanting, drumming, special objects, and movement create ritual, as does the creation of shrines and altars. The purpose of constructing thresholds (such as altars) that bring this world together is to find the powers that can heal the rends in tribal as well as modern com-

---

32. Bynum, "The African Origin of Familial Consciousness and the Dynamics of Dreaming."

munities.[33] Relations with ancestors can be maintained by honoring them at a shrine or altar, many of which are small and personal.

African spirituality embraces a life continuum that includes spiritual beings and ancestors. Ancestor reverence and healing traditions almost always include divination and dreams. Spiritual customs and healing practices are intertwined as integral aspects of a single cosmology. Both an understanding of dream imagery and knowledge of dream interpretation are essential in traditional African healing practices.[34] Dreams are an expression of personal, ancestral, and spiritual forces operating together through life and the body.

Later, the interjection of European colonialism onto African culture created a rupture in the philosophical underpinnings and the traditions. Many of the cultural, spiritual, and dream-sharing practices responded to this with a variety of adaptations, including Western Hemisphere variations such as Santeria and capoeira. These were created, at least in part, for the purpose of being able to continue to practice forbidden ancestral traditions "in plain sight."

In many African traditions, consciousness is seen as non-local—that is, not centered only in one's own body or mind, but shared more broadly. A shared dream can uplift a people, as Martin Luther King Jr.'s "I Have a Dream" speech still lifts hearts and holds visionary grandeur. Similarly, a shared nightmare, such as apocalyptic visions of the world, can create distress and fear. What starts as a personal dream can move into the collective unconscious, as it does in Carl Jung's collective unconscious.

Aboriginal Australian Dreaming

In classical Aboriginal Australian cosmology, ancestral beings are collectively held to have created the natural world and all that inhabit it. Here, where dreams are "at the very heart of cosmology, innovation, and social reproduction," there is an intimate relationship between dreams, perception, and creativity.[35] The unique cosmology of dreaming associated

---

33. Somé, *Ritual*.
34. Brewster, *Race and the Unconscious*, 374.
35. Tonkinson, *The Mardudjara Aborigines*.

with Australian Aboriginal cultures implies a fluidity of both form and consciousness between living people, animals, departed ancestors, gods, and the land itself. This concept is typically translated in English as the Dreaming, or sometimes as Dreamtime. The Dreaming represents the creation of everything: the time when the ancestral spirits moved across the land and created life as well as various landscape features. These beings and their substance and spirit remain an integral part of the topography of the land and sea. The Dreaming both creates and is created by the spirits of the people and the animals that walk the land.

Songlines

Paths across the land were drawn according to Songlines, walking routes that crossed the continent and told the stories of indigenous ancestors. The term *Songline* refers to the features and directions included in a song that had to be memorized and sung for a traveler to know the route to their destination. Certain Songlines were called "Dreaming Pathways" because these tracks were said to be forged by Creator Spirits during the Dreaming.[36] Many Songlines had specific ancestral stories attached to them. They have been called a "singing celebration" and are one way to recognize the footprints of the ancestors on the land.[37]

Before colonization, Songlines were maintained by regular use and clearing. Today, many have been paved over for general use by vehicles and modern municipalities.

Honoring Dreams

The general Aboriginal worldview contains an openness to interpretation. As with a dream, this worldview holds that multiple meanings are inherent or possible in any thing or event. For example, children grow up being intensely socialized into a world understood to be populated by ancestral beings. Children are regarded as especially sensitive to manifestations of ancestral presence if they have waking nocturnal visions in which they see

---

36. "Songlines."
37. "Songlines."

spirits of deceased relatives visiting. Great social value is placed on these visions.[38]

There is not a differentiation between waking or sleeping dream states or the information gathered from them. Ethnographic research across Australia shows that when tribal peoples experience dreams—and when ancestral beings, deceased relatives, and other spirits appear in these dreams—these experiences are understood as actual events that have occurred, not as something that happened "in the mind."[39] They are received as true experiences of one's spirit or soul.

Native American Ancestral Traditions and Dreams

As with many native and indigenous peoples, dreams and visions are considered a connection to the spiritual world and are an essential part of the wide range of Native American tribes and cultures. Here, too, dreams act as a bridge between the physical world and the spiritual one. Many tribal members practice dream incubation, trance states, shamanic journeying, and other forms of waking dreamwork to connect with their ancestors, to connect with the spirit world, and to receive guidance.

Protective dreamcatchers are hung over the beds of infants to catch or snare bad dreams and nightmares in their webbing, allowing good or pleasant dreams to slip through the hole in the center. Children are taught to remember their dreams from an early age, and tribal elders help them interpret the meanings. This deep spiritual connection through dreamwork also helps establish the respect and veneration of elders and ancestors.

In Native American tradition, creation is seen as a living process with kinship between all beings. Thus, as all the creators are family, acknowledging that they are our ancestors is said in gratitude. The Lakota phrase *Mitakuye Oyasin*, "all my relations," means all living things in the universe: The earth is our mother, the sky is our father, the rocks and trees and animals are our brothers and sisters, and all are sacred. The land itself

---

38. Eickelkamp, "Sand Storytelling," 113.
39. Tonkinson, *The Mardudjara Aborigines*.

is sacred. Thus, as all the creators are family, acknowledging that they are our ancestors is said in gratitude.

Colonization and the genocide of Native peoples created immeasurable traumas and a lasting displacement from Native spirituality, ritual, and tradition. Today, many young people are learning from their elders and re-embracing Native ritual, song, and language. However, there are still people who are unaware of Native ancestral connections. My colleague, Mia, learned as an adult that her grandfather six generations back had been the chief of the Oneida Nation; this was a secret that had been kept by Mia's father and his fathers before him. Then, Mia had the following dream that connected her with her Native heritage in a personal way:

> *I am in a village that feels foreign, as if from centuries ago, with thatched dwellings and dirt paths and people in Native American dress walking quietly about. I don't know where I am. I look for anything familiar but am increasingly distressed. I try to ask people where we are, but no one seems to hear me, and people act as if I'm just one of them. I begin to think I might be dead and start to panic. I know that somehow, I have to break out of this reality. Finally, in a burst of energy, I raise my fist and punch at the sky with all my might. I wake up, shaken and hugely relieved that this was "only" a dream.*

In this dream, Mia seems to have gone through a portal in time and space to return to a place where one of her ancestors lived. The tribe within which she landed in her dream seemed to notice nothing out of the ordinary in her being there with them. Mia herself became lucid in the dream (aware that she was dreaming within the dream itself) and realized that she was not in her proper time and place according to linear reality, and she panicked. She was then able to garner her strength and "punch at the sky with all [her] might" to break through the veil and return to the twenty-first century.

When Mia told me about this dream, she shared, "Since this dream, I have learned a great deal more about my family history. I now connect it to my decades-long passion for dream work. It may be that my ancestor the Chief was the dreamer for the tribe, as I tend to be gifted with precognitive dreams at times."[40]

This hidden or silenced piece of family history finally pierced the veil and found a willing and talented dreamer to be the memory keeper for the family. In contrast, as our Blackfoot guide took us through Glacier National Park in September 2024, he told us that he could trace and contact his living and deceased ancestors and descendants through six generations. His lineage had stayed a part of his family for six generations through dreams, artworks, and stories.

Navigating Dream Realms

The phrase *boundary skipping*, attributed to Shawn Wilson, speaks to the priority Native peoples place on the ability to traverse worlds.[41] Uncanny realms and non-linear ways of knowing are accessed through dreams, sweat lodge ceremonies, and other rituals, such as a solo vision quest.

Strong dreamers can travel to other worlds in dream states. For the Spokane tribe, there is the concept of three souls that can leave the body and travel in a form of astral projection during dreams and trance states to connect with ancestors, animal spirit guides, and guardian spirit guides. Anishinaabe peoples believe people have two souls, one of which travels at night and lives a dream in an alternate and valid reality. From this perspective, it is the soul that dreams, not the mind.

In many if not most Native American tribes, the shaman or medicine man or woman is chosen in large part because they are a strong dreamer who can use dreams to heal, teach, and unite people. They can dream and vision not only for themselves, but for the whole tribe. Prophetic dreamers then create action plans based on their dreams, such as planning for expected weather patterns, which may be interpreted by shamans. Many have also learned to control their dreams, similar to lucid dreaming in the modern world.

Dreams from many Native traditions are simply seen as reflections or mirrors of reality. In a study that included sixteen different tribes' approach

---

40. Mia Woodruff, email message to author, June 10, 2024.
41. Wilson, *Research Is Ceremony*.

to dreams, Krippner and Thompson write, "In most of the 16 Native American models, there is no distinct separation between the dreamed world and the lived world."[42] Therefore, we can surmise that the Native American perspective on dreams is that they essentially play the role of mirroring reality in the subconscious.

When three Abenaki members were interviewed in 2018, they confirmed that dreams are taken very seriously in their culture and have both a literal and symbolic meaning. Two interviewees confirmed that some dreams are visits from ancestors and are a way to understand and connect the past and the future.[43] The interviewer concludes, "Despite the victimization their people and culture faced from colonialism, their knowledge and traditions are passed on through dreams by connections with their ancestors. Dreaming thus is a form of resistance and preservation of their cultural identity."[44] Dreaming is part of the effort to keep Native traditions and history alive.

Ancestors and Dreaming in the Abrahamic Traditions and Texts

Many people don't realize that paying attention to dreams and the ancestors is also part of Jewish, Christian, and Islamic spiritual traditions and theology. These three faiths are called the Abrahamic traditions because they all share a common ancestor, the patriarch Abraham. The importance of dreams as a means of connecting with a divine source or wisdom, and making action plans to save or enhance life by attending to these dreams, threads its way through all three faiths. Joseph the dream interpreter is one of the better-known examples.

If you look at the Bible from Genesis on, you may be struck by how many of the chapters begin with or contain a litany of ancestors and descendants' names and progeny. Growing up, my family and friends called the long list of names in the Torah, the first five books of the Bible, "the begots." Abraham and Sarah begot Isaac, and Abraham and Hagar

---

42. Krippner and Thompson, "A 10-Facet Model of Dreaming," 94.
43. Casale, "Indigenous Dreams."
44. Casale, "Indigenous Dreams."

begot Ishmael (making Abraham the father of Islam as well as Judaism and Christianity). Isaac and Rebecca begot Jacob and Esau. Jacob and his two wives, Leah and Rachel, and their two handmaidens, Bilhah and Zilpah, begot the twelve named tribes and one daughter, Dinah. They are cited repeatedly throughout the Torah as the beginning of the ancestral legacy that leads through Jacob's twelve sons and one daughter, including Joseph, the dreamer, and on through Moses. The names of these elders continue to be invoked in subsequent texts. In Christian tradition, part of the acknowledgment of Jesus's importance derives from his connection to this ancestral line; he was a direct descendant of King David, from the tribe of Judah.

This naming of the ancestors and their descendants contributes to a sense of continuity with ancient and more immediate family history. The linear thread of ancestral connection can tell us where we come from, where we are going, and who we might become. Today, many families name their children after a relative to honor them and provide continuity in the family (i.e., James Jr.). In Jewish tradition, children aren't named for living relatives, but after the most recently departed family member as an honor to their memory. When someone dies, mourners say, "May their memory be for a blessing." If the name is unwieldy or too dated, sometimes the first letter of the departed's name is used instead, along with imparting the knowledge of the connection to the child. For example, "You, Becky, are named after your aunt Blanche." I never knew my great-uncle Louie, my grandma's brother, but all my life I have known that I am named after him. It is a part of my identity.

Desert Roots

The desert is raucously loud in its silence. The Middle East is largely desert, and it is where Jewish, Christian, and Muslim ancestors walked and lived. In the stillness of the desert, one can feel their soul-self with greater clarity, and if they sit quietly, it can become a soul-space where they can find peace and answers. Many prophets went out to the desert to receive visions and dreams. Sometimes visions or dreams came to the prophets while they were deep in a cave in the desert, adding another layer of seclusion. They came in the forms of nighttime dreams, of daytime visions, of a ladder connecting heaven and earth on which angels traveled up and down (Jacob), a burning bush that spoke (Moses), and in a still, small voice (Elijah). *Chalom* is the word meaning both dream and vision, and the context of the surrounding story can tell us if the messages came through in waking or sleeping time.

When there is not a lot of other distraction or noise, tuning in to dreams and visions becomes easier. In the luminous spaciousness of silence and stars, the ancestors heard and saw the messages of their dreams and visions more clearly.

Mystic Connections

Dreams and visions are part of history and mystical practice. The Talmud, which expands on the Torah, teaches that dreams are a gift and are one-sixtieth prophecy. It highlights the importance of understanding one's dreams, stating that a dream uninterpreted is like a letter unopened. People are further instructed to be careful to receive the understanding and interpretation of the dream that is true for them, since "all dreams follow the mouth," meaning that the manifestation of the dream in the waking world follows what one believes the dream meant.

Sufism is the mystical branch of Islam. In the Sufi system, divine word is often expressed through dreams and visions. Sufis believe that dreams are one-forty-sixth prophecy, a slight variation on the teachings of Talmud.

All three Abrahamic faiths have a similar bedtime prayer that asks the Divine to protect them in their sleep, gift them with true and good dreams, and have the sleeper wake up in peace and wholeness.

* * *

These are just a few of the many traditions that honor dreamwork and ancestral connections around the world. When we acknowledge and honor our shared ancestors and their teachings, we find that we have more in common than not. A good reminder for all of us in this fractured world.

Ancestors and Adoption

This unique family constellation deserves a section of its own to highlight the meaning of ancestry when adoption is part of your family. So, how do you acknowledge and explore ancestry when you yourself or a family member were adopted? There are several ways to attend to this, none of which are mutually exclusive.

First, there is no difference between the family status or the inheritance status of an adopted child and a biological child. If you have adopted a child, they are your child, period. Your relatives are their relatives; your family is their family. In addition to this, the adopted child has an additional biological family, also called a *birth family*. Some adoptees have no interest in exploring their biological roots, others are intensely interested, and everything in between. My friend Bob, who was adopted as an infant, said that when he was young, there was no forum for ancestral searches, and at this point in his life, it feels too far away and not important.

Talking to Your Child About Adoption

Never being told that you or a family member were adopted was a common pattern in previous generations, and it may still occur today. If this is/was the case, it then becomes a family secret. We know that secrets frequently surface at some point in time, and they are unnerving at best, maybe even traumatic. I believe it is a disservice to not tell an adopted child about their history. This could have a profound impact on their identity. Plus, their medical history becomes compromised if they think they share the genetics of their adopted family; my daughter simply writes "unknown" when medical forms ask her about her family health history.

The question of lineage often arises when a child is in elementary school and is asked to make a family tree. If they haven't yet been told about their history, this can create confusion or distress. If they are the same race and skin color as the adopting family, the question may not have arisen spontaneously; however, with multiracial adoption, it is immediately clear that the child has different biological roots and needs to know why they look different than their parents. Imagine discovering years down the road, or even generations later, that you are not who you thought you were. A shock at the very least, and it can raise questions about truthfulness and honesty in the family system. For many reasons, I encourage you to share their origin story with your adopted child, as best as you know it, and with as much or as little detail as is appropriate for their age. This helps to avoid uncomfortable encounters later on.

For very young children, start the conversation when they are old enough to understand (around age three, give or take, particularly if they don't look like you and questions have or could arise). It is enough to say you chose them to be their child. You might say something like, "We really wanted a child, and we chose you." Explain that they are part of your family, but they had a different birth mom and dad. At this stage, no details are needed about the actual biological creation of a child—that can come later.

As they get older, supply more information and details about their birth family and origin. Leave the door open for their curiosity and exploration. If you can, try to expose them to the traditions of their birth family. And, whatever your own family ancestry and traditions are, live them and pass them on to your children, however they joined your family.

My Daughter

One adoption anecdote I recall happened when my daughter was about three years old. She was sitting in the shopping cart seat while we walked around the grocery store. In one of the aisles, we were stopped by a woman who started asking all kinds of questions about foreign adoption. It bordered on inappropriate, and I endeavored to be polite but kept it brief. Afterward, I said to my daughter, "I'm so sorry, honey. I hope that wasn't too uncomfortable for you."

She replied, "Oh, Mommy, I was very uncomfortable."

Dismayed, I asked her what parts bothered her.

She replied, "We were standing in the freezer section of the store, and I was freezing! Couldn't she have asked in front of the cereal instead?"

Phew! Dodged a bullet on that one! Good reminder not to assume.

When my daughter was young, we connected with a local group of other families who had adopted children from China. We all met regularly for many years, sometimes just for play dates, but other times to learn Chinese calligraphy or some basic Chinese language. Together, we learned how to celebrate Chinese New Year.

When my daughter was ten years old, we traveled to China with a group. My daughter got to see the country of her birth and even visited the orphanage where she spent her first few months. The orphanage director and a "Hugging Granny"—a surrogate grandmother from the neighboring senior home—were both there when she was an infant, and they still remembered her. She was warmly welcomed. It was a powerful and moving experience for all of us, and it became the equivalent of meeting long-lost family members.

My daughter remained interested in her biological origins throughout her teen years, which we supported. For her eighteenth birthday, we bought her a kit from 23andMe, a company that does genetic testing and ancestry composition via saliva samples. After she submitted her saliva sample, she got some information about her biological history that was fascinating to her, but there were no connections to any family members.

When my daughter was in her early twenties, she was contacted out of the blue by a woman in California. The woman said that it seemed my daughter was related to her adopted daughter, who was about eight years old at the time; the genetic tracing from 23andMe indicated that their great-grandmothers were sisters. This biological connection has meant a great deal to my daughter and enhanced her own origin story. The girls have been in touch ever since and are planning a visit.

Orienting the Next Generation to Dream Power

Culture and experience shape dream content and how dreams are received. How might the world be different if all children were raised to value sleeping and waking dreamtime and dream encounters? As I mentioned in chapter 1, I am so glad I introduced my own daughter to this worldview before she was old enough to question it or think it was weird.

Think about how you could orient the next generation to the power of dreams and dreaming. You might wish to journal about this for posterity. Spend a few moments crafting how you would explain the connection between worlds to a child. Think about the age and developmental life stage of kiddos you know and frame it accordingly. How would you explain why dreams are important? How might you explain ancestors to them? How might you explain what it means if an ancestor visits their dreams? How do you want to orient your young to the value of non-linear ways of knowing?

Creating Your Own Ancestral Dreaming Traditions

Take some time to acknowledge and to learn about your own history and traditions in the worlds of dreamtime and ancestral connections. Where is your family from? How far back can you trace your lineage? Go back to your genogram and fill in countries of origin if you haven't already. Are there already practices in your family tradition that are perpetuated from generation to generation and/or connected to ethnic, cultural, or tribal traditions? Did parts of your family originate in Ireland, or Italy, or Haiti? Or do you trace family history to China, or Ukraine, or Egypt? What are the traditions in your family around acknowledging ancestors? Do you acknowledge the anniversaries of a death, and if so, for how long? Are you lucky enough to have relatives still alive who can fill in some blanks for you? Don't wait too long to ask.

Ancestor Altars and Additional Ways to Honor Your Ancestors

You can create an altar or memory place in your bedroom or another part of your home to both honor your loved ones and to invite them into your dreams. This can serve as a place to make contact and encourage their connection, advice, wisdom, or mutual healing.

The altar can hold pictures, artifacts, things of beauty, candles, incense, bells, or gongs; feel free to add anything that allows all your senses to engage with honoring and accessing your ancestors. Mine has pictures, shells, crystals, a pair of small white doves, a cat statue (we consider cats to be family members), a small urn of some of my grandmother's ashes, and icons or markers of all the cultures our extended family embraces.

Sometimes loved ones will just show up in your dreams or in waking-life synchronicities, but if you make a place for them to feel welcome, they may be more likely to feel your intention. As I am writing this, I wonder if part of the reason my dad is such a frequent flier in my dreams is because I have a picture of him as part of the little altar I have on my dresser.

In addition to altars, you are honoring and opening space for your ancestors when you use their holiday dishes, make their traditional foods, or hang the pictures that adorned their walls on your own walls after they have passed. You can choose to honor them purposefully by doing these small rituals with intentionality.

You may also inherit family heirlooms. Sometimes they are religious or spiritual items, like Mom's rosary or Dad's tallit (prayer shawl). You can choose to use heirlooms or to simply acknowledge them if they are not your custom anymore. For example, my mother-in-law was a devoted follower of Swami Chinmayananda Saraswati, a Hindu holy man. In her lifetime she collected multiple statues and pictures of this spiritual path. After she passed last year, many of them migrated over to our house as my husband honored his mother, her beliefs, and her taste in art. They now mingle with the pictures and artifacts that honor our daughter's Chinese heritage and ancestry as well our Seder plate, menorah, and candlesticks.

FIVE

GRIEFWORK AND ANCESTORS

> Each day at hospice
> The cat adopts a soul
> It purrs to final rest.
> —*Mia Woodford*

The band Maroon 5 has a song titled "Memories." It is about remembering loved ones who have passed on as they toast their memory by raising a glass. When I first heard the song, I heard a line from the chorus and thought that they sang about the dreams bringing back all the memories; I later discovered I misheard the lyrics, and the word is *drinks*, not *dreams*! While drinks may also help us bring back memories and recall our ancestors, I know that my personal Freudian slip interpretation is also correct. Dreams *do* bring back memories, maybe even better than drinks. To this day, I continue to sing along with the chorus using my own word, both because that is what I already had internalized and because I get a kick out of it.

Various Connections with the Departed

Rabbi Irwin Keller writes that his mother used to laugh and say to him, "Be careful, I might come back and haunt you."[45] He writes about noticing that his laugh sounds like his mother's, and some of the expressions he makes on his face match his mother's particular expressions. Keller

---

45. Keller, "In These Last Months of 2023, I Have Noticed the Jewish Ancestors in Me More than Ever."

acknowledges that these expressions have their own origin, not just in his mother, but in generations past, saying, "We carry the ancestors in us. We carry them in a vast mosaic of talents and traits and traumas."[46] As he honors the anniversary of his mother's death each year, Keller notes the long legacy of ancestors he and his mother carry: the gifts and the troubles, the whispers of love and the shouts of pain.

Family legacies, both of love and of pain, can move backward and forward in time, like dreams themselves. As I shared in chapter 1, over half of all Americans connect with their departed loved ones, mostly through their dreams. Departed loved ones may seek your attention—or you may seek theirs—through spontaneous dreams and nighttime visitations, through a request for contact with an incubated dream, through synchronistic experiences, or through waking "dreamish" occurrences. Often, a sweet or bitter visit from your ancestors corresponds with the work of grieving: grieving that needs to occur so healing can happen on many realms.

Stages of Grief

When you grieve a loss, the process may be simple and uncomplicated, or it may be complex and multifaceted. Uncomplicated loss of a beloved is sad: You may mourn, cry, wail, and miss them, but you are generally not left with feelings of intense anger, pain, or anxiety that feel larger than life.

Anger is a normal part of the grieving process. In 1969, Elisabeth Kübler-Ross famously delineated five stages of grief in her seminal book *On Death and Dying*: denial, anger, bargaining, depression, and resolution or acceptance. These phases are often spoken of as if they are linear, but in fact, they come and go. Kübler-Ross later spoke out about how these stages were misinterpreted as linear and integrated them into her Change Curve.[47]

The stages of grief are more like a spiral and can repeat for the first year or two following a significant loss. During the first year after a death, it is

---

46. Keller, "In These Last Months of 2023, I Have Noticed the Jewish Ancestors in Me More than Ever."
47. "Kübler-Ross Change Curve."

the first of everything without them: the first birthday, the first Thanksgiving, etc. The second year after a loss is given short shrift in Western society, but it can contain powerful memories and triggers as we more fully adjust to life without a loved one.

Denial

The stage of denial often includes feeling numb or in shock as your system tries to make sense of your new reality. Denial protects you from becoming completely overwhelmed. You may find yourself saying things like "I can't believe it" or "I keep expecting them to be in the next room." Often, it is like you have partially shut down. In some ways, denial is like the process of dissociation, which also serves to protect you. You may need a bit of distance from the loss, whether or not it was expected.

As you move through the stage of denial, you may start to notice the presence of your loved one, either through a felt sense, hearing their voice, or seeing them in your dreams. This can be a sign of movement toward a gradual acceptance of the loss.

Anger

Anger is a normal response to loss. Loss can feel unfair, especially if someone died young or tragically, or if you had plans with that person that now can't be carried out. You might feel angry that they died and thus deprived you of their company, or you might be angry with yourself for things you didn't do or say before they passed. You may also be angry at caregivers or medical professionals if you feel they didn't do the right thing. Know that it is not too late to continue to connect and converse.

Bargaining

When you have lost a loved one, it can be hard to accept that there is nothing you can do to bring them back. You might try to make deals with yourself or with the Divine in the hopes that if you do certain things or act in certain ways, it will mitigate your pain or loss. You might find yourself thinking *What if…*or *If only…*

I was able to bypass the bargaining stage of grief by listening to my inner voice. Before my mom died, she suddenly got very sick and was rushed to the hospital with organ failure; I knew it was serious from the description her friend gave me. While we were both originally from Buffalo, my mom was in Florida for the winter, and I live in Boston. I am eternally grateful that I had the wherewithal to hop on a plane a day later. When one of my siblings asked why I was going, since there wasn't anything we could actually do, I replied, "Just to be with her."

I spent the weekend in Florida, going back and forth from my mom's condo to the hospital. I hung out, gave my mom neck massages, brought her sweet treats (her weakness), gifted flowers to the nursing staff, and befriended the doctor. It turned out that he was from Buffalo originally too! I am convinced he gave my mother some extra TLC because of our Buffalo connection.

My mom was stable when I left on Sunday with a heavy heart. I said, "We'll be in touch. See you soon."

As I was driving to the airport, I heard out loud what I believe was a spirit voice, just as if it was in the car with me. That voice sounded like me telling my brothers, "Mom died." One day later, she did.

What layer on the continuum of consciousness was that voice? Probably somewhere between reverie, synchronicity, and spontaneous trance. Now, whenever I question whether or not I should truly trust my inner voice, I remember when I encountered it telling me to go to Florida to be with my mom, and then it prepared me for her death. So, no regrets. In this way, I was able to bypass the bargaining stage of grief after my mom's death.

Depression

The sadness you feel after a loss can manifest as depression, with all the physical and emotional symptoms that often accompany it: lethargy, loss of appetite, joylessness, withdrawal from the company of others, longing, and feeling that life no longer has meaning. It is normal for these feelings to come and go over many months. As long as these symptoms do not persist more than a few months, they are likely part of the normal process of grieving. If symptoms persist, or if they are interfering with your ability to connect with others and the activities of your own life, it may be time to seek professional help. Grief groups can be particularly helpful for those in this stage of grief. Being with others helps humans process loss, so try to stay connected to community, even if it is hard. At our core, people are relational beings, so we often find the most healing when we are surrounded by others.

Resolution/Acceptance

In this stage of grief, you no longer are in denial, even though you may wish the death hadn't happened. You accept the reality of your loved one's passing and figure out how to move on in life without their physical presence. You may reconnect with aspects of day-to-day life, though waves of grief will still wash over you from time to time. Especially if you have lost someone precious or close to you, you don't "get over" a loss, but you learn to live again, perhaps raising a drink (or a dream!) to their memory from time to time. If you are in touch with your loved one between worlds, you generally have a loving encounter that feeds your soul and reaffirms your connection, rather than an encounter that causes pain, guilt, or upset.

Last fall, I was writing while traveling through the Canadian Rockies. When a fellow traveler on the train learned what I was writing about, she told me that she had been afraid of death after her sister, brother-in-law, and husband all died within a year of each other. A year later, she had a waking dream/vision that she was holding Jesus's hand. He was dressed all in white, and her sister as a young child came skipping up to greet her with a big bouquet of flowers. Then her husband called out to her from a nearby park bench, saying, "Come and sit down. I can answer your questions." She told me that has not feared death since she had this dream.

When you can turn your grief into some form of beauty and connection, you are well on your way to acceptance, moving on, and honoring the life of your departed loved ones.

Bereavement Dreams

Dreams of the deceased tend to ease the process of grieving, as many of these dreams offer messages of comfort and assurance. Bereavement dreams appear to serve at least three distinct functions: They can assist with processing trauma; they can serve to maintain a bond with the deceased; and/or they can help regulate emotion. Taken together, these functions may "actively facilitate adjustment to bereavement."[48]

Poet Martín Prechtel tells us that our grief is praise for the departed; it is a sacred art. Some people rush to "get over" grief because they see it as a weakness, as hanging on to loss, but Prechtel feels grief is really hanging on to love, which is why we always feel it.[49] There is a difference between painful, heart-rending loss and the bittersweet loss of remembering a beloved. When the initial shock and pain of the loss have been worn smoother with the sands of time, we can remember a deceased loved one with fondness and warmth.

With that being said, some bereavement dreams are distressing. This is often the case when the relationship with the departed was difficult. When this is the case, bereavement dreams fall into numbers four and five of the types of ancestor dreaming outlined in chapter 1: The deceased experienced pain or trauma in their life and are coming to you to ask for help and healing ("Please, please help and heal me; I am still suffering"), or they are stuck on a vendetta that may have begun years or even centuries before ("Watch out: This old grudge has not yet been resolved").

Bereavement dreams may also be distressing if you yourself have unfinished business with the departed. Bad blood may continue to haunt you if they died before an argument, disagreement, or estrangement could be resolved. Another example that shows up more often than you might expect is an inheritance conflict after someone's death; there may be painful, heartbreaking, or vicious arguments about the deceased's will or an inheritance. Or, for some other reason, you may be unable to let them go. This type of attachment is different than finding comfort and solace in the departed's presence; it is more about your need to hang on in a way that no longer serves you. These types of dream themes are what Alcoholics Anonymous call the "woulda, coulda, shoulda" thoughts and feelings, or the "if only" reflections.

There is also the case of a tangled spirit. In these instances, the spirit of a loved one has become inexplicably caught between worlds, tangled up

---

48. Ellis, "Dreams of Bereavement."
49. Prechtel, *The Smell of Rain on Dust*, 5, 31.

in the in-between, or the bardo space. The numerous translations of the Tibetan Book of the Dead speak of the bardo as the indeterminate space between the living and the dead. In this space, the consciousness of the dead can still hear and comprehend the prayers and words of the living spoken on the dead's behalf, which can help the dead navigate through confusion and finish their passage to the other side.[50]

I encourage you to check your soul-consciousness to see if you can help tangled spirits, and if your work is to bless them and help send them all the way over. If you have not contributed to the tangles in time and space, then perhaps you need a ritual to help them cross over.

EXERCISE
Helping Tangled Spirits Over the Threshold

If tangled spirits or over-attachments are keeping your ancestors stuck in the in-between, try this waking exercise. (Note: If it is pain or unhealed trauma keeping tangled spirits stuck, you will learn how to work with them in chapter 8.)

1. Surround yourself with a blue container of light, or whatever color(s) allows you to have strong, clear boundaries between the world of the living and the world of the dead. Allow this container to be clear enough that you can communicate through it easily, but strong enough that neither side of the veil permeates the other.

2. Once you are aware that they have contacted you, whether it was through your dreams or in waking life, you can ask these ancestors what is keeping them in limbo. Listen carefully to discern if you have any part in keeping their spirit or essence too close to the world of the living, or if they have simply lost their way or become disoriented in their passage to the beyond.

3. If you realize that you have a part in the spirit's inability to move on (for example, they may say something

---

50. Rinpoche, *The Tibetan Book of Living and Dying*.

like "Don't go, I can't bear it! Don't leave me"), offer them your version of this blessing or prayer:

Dearest ancestor or loved one,

I now release you from all unnecessary attachments to the world of the living. I apologize if I have inadvertently participated in keeping you from completing your journey to the other side and your transition to the world of spirit. I will do my part and seek out what I need for my own healing in this world and release all parts of you to reside with the One. I promise that we will continue to connect in love once you have finished your transition to your new home. We will then find a way we can offer each other comfort from that place.

May it be so.

4. If the spirit is not held back by any over-attachment on your part, but has simply become disoriented, offer them your version of the following blessing:

Dearest ancestor or loved one,

It is now time for you to complete your journey home. Turn to the light. See the shining palace that your soul can reside in. Your work here is done. Become oriented and clear on your path. See the path of shining brightness before you, calling you in the right direction, calling you home.

Step forward and complete your journey now.

May it be so.

5. After speaking your blessing, take a deep breath. Blow out a *whoosh* sound as you exhale, adding your soul-breath to help them along. You could also add some movement, such as lifting your hands or arms in the direction the departed needs to travel, usually upward. Do this three times or until you sense when the spirit has moved on.

* * *

I love this quote by John O'Donohue.

> *The dead are not distant or absent. They are alongside us. When we lose someone to death, we lose their physical image and presence, they slip out of visible form into invisible presence. This alteration of form is the reason we cannot see the dead. But because we cannot see them does not mean that they are not there. Transfigured into eternal form, the dead cannot reverse the journey and even for one second re-enter their old form to linger with us a while. Though they cannot reappear, they continue to be near us and part of the healing of grief is the refinement of our hearts whereby we come to sense their loving nearness.*[51]

I love this concept of alteration of form. It lends poetic credence to the felt sense of the deceased's ongoing presence among the living. The quality of "lifefullness" that is contained in the physical body—called the soul by many—is the part that does not die when the human body does. Sometimes the form of the dead remains in your consciousness or waking sphere, but other times they only come through when your conscious self is off duty enough to let them in, which happens when you sleep and dream.

Complicated and Uncomplicated Grief

It is important to note that physical discomfort, pain, and distress following trauma or tragic loss are not just "all in your head." Oftentimes, people feel their feelings emotionally and physically. No one ever just "gets over" a significant loss; it may remain a hole in your life for years to come. However, there are several kinds of grief you may experience.

Complicated Grief

Complicated grief may occur if the departed was an addict, mentally ill, or overtly narcissistic; this can lead to a different kind of loss. If you were hurt physically, emotionally, or sexually by the departed, their death may

---

51. O'Donohue, *Beauty*.

become a muddled and ambiguous combination of grief and relief. Complicated grief also arises when the departed was abusive, neglectful, or had dysfunctional behaviors that contributed to an unsafe family home. If your family looked perfectly intact from the outside (pillars of the community, as it were) and the harm done behind closed doors was kept a secret from the world for various reasons such as fear, threat, or shame, then you may find yourself in a double bind after a family member's death. It can be challenging to respond to condolences when you are also thinking, *If you only knew who they really were...*

Complicated grief and/or tragic loss takes an additional toll on the survivor and can reach its long, sticky fingers down generational paths.

Uncomplicated Grief

If you had a good relationship with a departed ancestor—one not fraught with tension or abuse or abandonment—then the grieving process is more straightforward. You will miss them, be sad, talk about them with others, go through mourning rituals, and gradually resume your everyday life. As time goes on, you will recall your ancestors fondly, keep pictures of them around, and create a new normal without their physical presence. You may tell stories of their life or reference them in conversations with others long after they have passed. They remain with you, albeit in spirit rather than body.

There are times, however, when it is not that easy. Part of the mourning process involves talking about deceased loved one and sharing memories. When that does not happen for various reasons, individuals can get stuck in unprocessed grief. Perhaps you were not able to attend a funeral or celebration of life. You may need to do something later to get closure.

When I was in my early twenties, my dad died. I was living in Israel, and a giant January snowstorm in Buffalo, New York, prevented me from being able to go home for his funeral. I recall getting the phone call that he had died and the feeling of disbelief as the initial denial and numbness hit me. I had nowhere to go, no action steps I could take, and no ability to connect with others who were also mourning him. (This was way before Zoom was an option.) So, I just walked around the village I was living in with my roommate. I remember holding a cup of coffee in my hand as we walked and talked. She had lost both of her parents as a teen, and I recall feeling that I didn't want to upset her and talk about my dad too much in case it was hard for her. I held back some of what I might have said to take care of her feelings. In retrospect, I could have just asked her if it was okay to go into more detail, but in my early twenties, I didn't think about asking. That was it, my whole grieving ritual. Later that year, in the summer, I returned to the states and was able to visit the grave with my brothers to get a better sense of closure. Years later, I recognized that there were parts of my dad's life and death that were still haunting me, and I worked through some additional layers of grief and healing in my own therapy.

Ambiguous Loss

In addition to complicated and uncomplicated grief is the grief that accompanies ambiguous loss. A death is clear cut in some ways, and a divorce is generally final. But what about grief that is not acknowledged by society, or loss that is unclear or ambiguous in some way? For example, consider a beloved who lies between life and death, perhaps in a coma, or who suffered a stroke and cannot communicate. There is ongoing grief here, an incomplete mourning process. There is a sense of loss when a loved one has dementia, even if they are still alive. Ambiguous loss may also accompany the loss after a stillbirth, miscarriage, or abortion. Western society doesn't provide us with ready-made rituals for these kinds of losses. In cases such as these, it's possible that no one even knows about the ambiguous loss or the toll it is taking on the griever. But humans heal better in companionship, so it may be time to develop rituals that honor ambiguous loss too. These losses are also a part of your story.

Even with a joyous change, there can be ambiguous, unnamed loss. If you are preparing to marry your beloved, you may be celebrating while mourning the loss of your single life and the kind of freedom that comes with that. If you got the job you really wanted but need to move to take it, you may be excited while feeling sad about moving away from family. These are losses too, even more so if one of your relatives is ill or near death.

Chapter Five

Family Secrets and Shutdowns

Complicated family dynamics can lead to generational dysfunction. If the departed engaged in guilt-tripping such as "I sacrificed so much for you. You should be grateful," your legacy burden may be similar to the concept of "gifts with teeth": There are family obligations and loyalty binds that you seem to have inherited and feel a need to repay, although you don't know why.

What you know about the departed *and* what you don't know can affect you, as you learned in chapter 3. Secrets can create their own wounds, and the effort of burying information—even if you are not consciously aware of it—takes a toll and saps your energy and life force. What is not processed can surreptitiously show up in later generations. If you don't metabolize it, you run the chance of metastasizing it.

In her research, Dr. Rachel Yehuda found that the children and grandchildren of survivors of trauma had nightmares of being chased, freezing cold, forced to march over rough terrain, and imprisoned.[52] These were their ancestors' experiences, not their own, but they were dreaming about these experiences nonetheless. In many cases, the dreamer's parents and grandparents had not told anyone about their experiences. After surviving abuse, torture, trauma, or tragic loss, there is an understandable tendency to want to shut it away, to move on and not talk about it. This can be true in spades when a whole culture or community has been subject to loss or annihilation. Unfortunately, the past doesn't cooperate with the survivor's wishes and desires, and it will re-emerge at some point in time to be dealt with, if not in one generation, then in another.

I have shared that there is a difference between dwelling in the past and processing the past. This is key. Communities need grieving rituals just as much as individuals. In this way, the past is honored rather than buried, preventing it from emerging as a nightmare or dysfunction in subsequent generations.

Events do not have to be traumatic to cause a family to shut down. Oftentimes in families, the dead are quickly buried and not talked about.

---

52. Yehuda and Lehrner, "Intergenerational Transmission of Trauma Effects."

Silence buries but does not resolve a loss. There may have been shame or embarrassment connected to someone's life or death, such as suicide, family cut-offs and unhealed estrangements, inheritances or other financial disagreements, illegal activities, or abuse. Situations of untimely death, such as the loss of a child, may also cause a family to shut down, especially if the family has no support system or is given questionable advice. This is what happened in Shoshana's family.

The Path to Healing a Family Secret

This is a powerful example of how a secret loss and buried grief affected multiple generations of a family, and how that family finally found healing and closure.

Lynn was described as "beautiful, vivacious, and charismatic." Tragically, she died of kidney failure in 1961, when she was just fourteen. At the time, Lynn's brother, Joel, was ten, and their other brother was seventeen. Both boys were traumatized by the loss of their sister, but in 1961 there was little, if any, support for grieving families. When reflecting on that period of his life, Joel said that finding their peace with grief was not possible. Lynn's pictures came down. Slowly, all signs of her were removed from the house or stored in the attic. Joel said that the boys gave comfort to their mother, gave space to their father, and never spoke of their sister. The silence of Lynn's absence was deafening. The surviving siblings were overlooked, and Joel had to learn to suppress the pain of this tremendous loss.

After consulting their rabbi, Joel's parents took his advice and had another child, whom they named Ron. Ron was born just one year after Lynn's death, into the family's secret grief. Hard as it may be to imagine now, Joel's parents did not tell Ron about Lynn, and they did not want anyone else to do so either. When he was ten years old, Ron found a box of get-well cards and letters in a dusty box in the attic. That is how he discovered the sister he never knew he had. Because Joel's parents could not talk about Lynn, silence descended once again as the family lived with Lynn's ghost.

Chapter Five

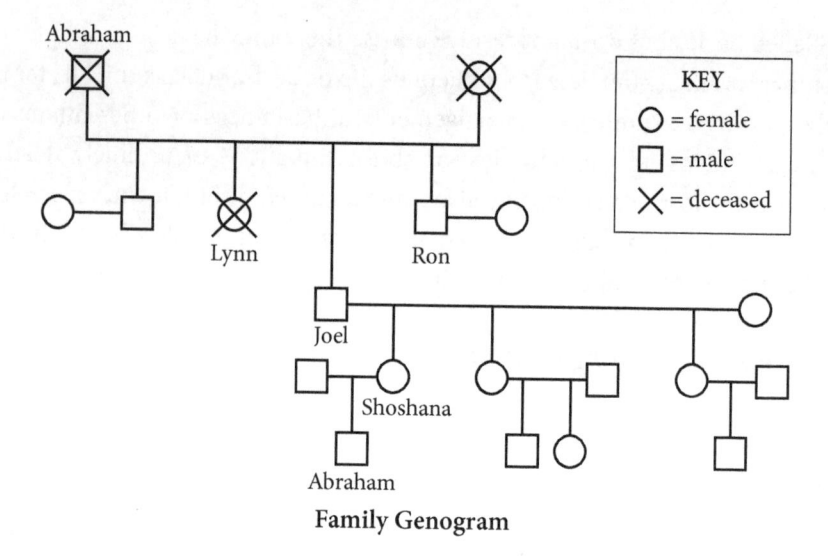

Family Genogram

In adulthood, Joel and his brother made attempts to resurrect Lynn's memory within the family. However, their parents resisted. When his mother was in her eighties, Joel asked her why she couldn't talk about Lynn. She told him that she was afraid if she started crying, she would never be able to stop.

Joel went on to have a family of his own, including a daughter named Shoshana. Shoshana learned about Aunt Lynn when her parents thought she was old enough to comprehend the story, around age eight or nine. Eventually, Shoshana became a mother herself, making Joel a grandfather. She named her son Abraham after his great-grandfather.

Finally, fifty-six years after Lynn's death, with the "gentle prodding of the next generation," the family decided to establish a memorial award in Lynn's honor. Joel's family was ready to bring Lynn back into their family and fulfill the mitzvah of honoring the dead.

A few days before the award ceremony, Shoshana had the following dream. At the time of her dream, baby Abraham was just a few months old.

> *I am standing at the front door of an unfamiliar house, but I know I am there to celebrate something. I don't know what. I ring the bell, and a pale boy who looks to be twelve or thirteen answers the door. He has*

sparkling green eyes, freckles, and curly brown hair. He is full of life and joy and ease.

"Hello!" he says. "You must be here for Lynn's ninetieth birthday party."

I peer over his shoulder and can see that the house is filled with happy, bustling people. Many of them look like family to me, but I don't recognize their faces. I can sense very strongly that Aunt Lynn is in an inner room of the house, holding court at her birthday party.

The boy keeps talking to me. "I'm Abe," he says. "In your world, my grandma died when she was fourteen. But in my world, she survived."

I want to meet Lynn but somehow know I can't. Still, I am filled with a sense of joy and completion.

Shoshana went on to say, "The dream was stunningly real. It feels less like I dreamed than like I got to glimpse through a portal between worlds. I have clearly met this world in the 'future' since Lynn would have been about seventy at the time I dreamed it. But the boy in my dream, like my son, is named after Lynn's and my dad's father, Abraham."[53]

This family resolved the pain generated by secret silence, silence that kept their grief buried and frozen, by moving forward and backward in time. Not only did Lynn's family honor their sister/aunt with an award in her honor, but Shoshana dreamed forward in time to a parallel universe in which her son met his aunt and celebrated her never-achieved birthday. Family legacies, like dreams themselves, can move forward and backward in time as well. At the time of this writing, Shoshana's son is about seven years old and has had some developmental challenges. In her dream, however, her son is twelve or thirteen and is a bright-eyed child full of ease, his challenges met and resolved. May it be so.

We can safely say that Lynn has now been put to a peaceful rest, and her name is remembered. Establishing a fund or scholarship in a loved one's name is a great way to answer the sixth ancestral call. ("Carry on my name and gifts to your children and your children's children. Remember.")

---

53. Shoshana Friedman, email message to author, January 11, 2024.

It is a special blessing both for the departed and for their family, as it keeps someone's memory alive.

At the time of Lynn's death, in the early 1960s, the importance of recognizing and naming the dead was not part of the culture. Ron, who was born after his sister's death but was never even told about her, carried the additional burden of being the only one who did not know, the only one who bore the secret.

Families frequently project their unfilled hopes and dreams for a child who died onto the next child born. This pattern can create the burden of living up to these expectations. Projections can unconsciously be passed on to subsequent generations via epigenetics, contributing to generational wounds.

How, Then, Do We Grieve?

Family members of different ages and generations often have different relationships to the pain of the past. The survivors—those who experienced the loss or atrocity personally—still held their pain close to the surface. Sometimes, this pain functioned as a scar or wound, but other times it was invisible to the eye and others were not aware of it. In the case of an invisible wound, the mourner would never be invited to talk about their grief. And if they didn't talk about it, they could pretend it didn't happen.

The next generation—the descendants of the survivors—wanted to move on, to forget, both what they knew and what they didn't quite know but sensed. Often, they just didn't ask. They learned this style of coping from their parents, who seemed to personify the phrase "Don't ask, don't tell." As one adult told me, the message she got from her father was, "Dead is dead."

However, subsequent generations (like the third and fourth generations, who had more distance from the survivor) often wanted to dig, to uncover, to talk about it. They then became the memory keepers for the family, hopefully asking for details before the survivors passed and were no longer available to verify them.

Exodus 34:7 says that the missteps or errors of each generation are passed down to the third and fourth generations. Whether we take this literally or not, you learned in chapter 3 that women epigenetically carry the seeds of the third or fourth generation within them. The message here is to keep talking and keep remembering. Learn the stories of your ancestors so you can be aware of the past. Decide which stories you want to pass down intact, with no change in the messaging, and which stories you want to transform for the purpose of healing. Intergenerational storytelling will help you reflect on memory and identity, both of which are crucial for recalling the past, understanding the present, and healing the future.

A theme threaded through the book *When the Body Says No* is that healing doesn't come from suppression—it comes from expression.[54] So, how can you express your grief and honor your ancestors? Consider gravestones, altars, touchstones, memory keepers, pictures, memorials, scholarship funds, talismans, and amulets. Integrate something concrete that allows you to touch, see, and name those who have gone before you. This puts their spirit to rest *and* keeps their name and memory alive. In this way, you can keep their spirit and good work going and/or put an end to their pain so they—and you!—can move forward in peace.

Amulets of Time

You could also honor your ancestors with "amulets of time," a phrase used by author James Runcie. Amulets of time are the small daily pleasures you can bookmark in your mind and come back to: the trill of a lark, the site of the first green shoot that pokes up in the spring, the open arms of the friend you haven't seen in a long time. Sometimes you will get a frisson of déjà vu when encountering an amulet of time, a sense of a synchronicity in time and/or space; this may be a glimpse of the memory of a Bright One in your lineage. It then becomes a touchstone whenever you see or experience this sight or event.

My friend Becka lost her father a few months ago. He loved sailing and whales and had even named his sailboats *Orca* and *Beluga*. Shortly after his death, Becka and her brother went sailing and saw a large pod of whales. One of them breached, completely out of the water, and she felt sure that was a sign from their dad. No doubt this will be an amulet in time for her.

---

54. Maté, *When the Body Says No*.

Cardinals are an amulet in time for me. Whenever I see them, I feel my stepfather, Bud, with me. My mother's necklace of small, multicolored glass beads is an amulet of time as well. I save it for special occasions and "dressing up." Whenever I get a compliment on it (almost every time I wear it), I get to say with a smile, "It was my mother's." I feel a sense of extra warmth and pride. My mother's necklace is an amulet in time and in relationship.

EXERCISE
Recognizing and Discerning Your Ancestors

Before beginning this exercise, surround yourself with a blue container of light for safety and protection. Keep the boundaries between yourself and others intact in all worlds.

1. Close your eyes. Feel the fullness of your own being, complete and whole. Once you are grounded and protected, sense or notice if any ancestors are swirling around or trying to break through your boundaries.

2. Tune in to your felt senses. Has anyone shown up and declared themselves an ancestor that you don't recognize? Ask for their name and listen. If you can, ascertain who they are and how they are connected to you: Are they a sibling, great-aunt, or distant great-great-great-grandfather?

3. Next, ask your ancestors what they need, what they want, and if you can help them find peace. An ancestor's request may be as simple as remembering their name and telling your children, or more may be needed. Their life, including their accomplishments and sufferings, may need to be honored and shared as well. Do they need an endowment in their name, a plaque in a place of worship, a gravestone, or a tree planted in their honor? Do they need a relative to be named after them? Would they like a prayer or blessing recited? Would they like you to create an altar in their memory inside or outside your home? This is of course a

partial list; you may have additional ideas. Pay attention to the answers you receive.

4. Take a deep breath, open your eyes, and gently wiggle your body to fully come back into the room. Then pick up your journal (or computer) and write down what you received intuitively. Before you finish writing, craft a plan to honor your ancestor's request, or at least craft the beginning stages of an action plan.

In this way, you can bring peace and connection forward and backward in the infinity of time and space, honoring the ones who came before and the ones who will come after. Blessings on their names.

* * *

I read an article about a young man who had lived through and lost relatives in war. I can no longer find the article link, but I remember what he wrote because it touched me. The young man believed that after a person passes, their soul is collected to the larger bundle of life. He felt that the soul works from many places, particularly for the relatives of the dead, and that when we face difficulties in life, the souls of our loved ones continue to act behind the scenes for us. He believed the dead do not leave us; they are watching us, happy about our joys and sharing in our sorrows. Last, he believed the dead are proud of us.

SIX

THE EMBODIED NATURE OF TRAUMA, NIGHTMARES, AND INTERGENERATIONAL TRAUMA TRANSMISSION

> The body is where we live, and where we first respond.
> —*Resmaa Menakem, My Grandmother's Hands*

When my dreamers or my clients bring in a dream or nightmare, some of the questions I typically ask are "What is your felt sense in your body right now? Just notice that to start with. Sit with it and see what happens next," and "Where in your body do you feel that? What is the physical sensation there in that spot? How would you describe it? What are the emotions that go with that sensation? How intense are they, on a scale of zero to ten?"

Two other lines of questioning that frequently yield paydirt are "What is the youngest part of you that is in the room right now that has experienced this?" and/or "Where in your family line did this begin? It doesn't matter if you know for sure—what does your gut sense or your intuition tell you?"

Treating intergenerational trauma from an embodied perspective is based on the work of many practitioners and scholars. We can thank mind/body practitioners and scholars Bessel van der Kolk, Babette Rothschild, Peter Levine, Pat Ogden, Bert Hellinger, Gabor Maté, Resmaa Menakem, Mark Wolynn, and Stephen Porges. For image-specific and embodied work in the dreaming world, we rest on the shoulders of dream experts Stephen Aizenstat, Robert Bosnak, Jean Campbell, Robert Hoss, Arnold Mindell, Catherine Shainberg, Jeremy Taylor, Eugene Gendlin, and of course Carl Jung.

When considering all the research that has been done on the mind/body connection and dreamwork, body-based dreaming takes on new significance. Let's start with an example of body-based dreaming that was about an embrace.

Healing in Company

My colleague Johanna lost her beloved father, Peter, after a twelve-year battle with cancer. Prior to Peter's death, Johanna had several visitation dreams, which she felt helped prepare her for his passing. Since then, she has been comforted by the presence of others both in her waking life and in her dreams. On her father's birthday, Johanna had the following dream.

> *There is a farewell party in my father's apartment. Many people, many children, including my daughter, her husband, my granddaughters, and a newborn baby. I have pain in the heart chakra at the back. A man called Peter (which is my father's name as well!) from the Holotropic Breathwork team offers me a session.*[55]

> *We lie embraced in the room next to the kitchen surrounded by lots of people.... We lie there on the floor, completely relaxed, in the middle of the hustle and bustle. I tell Peter that my second husband had just left the party and said goodbye, and I also tell him about my first husband, who died twelve years ago. My third husband is also here, but nevertheless, I enjoy the flow of unconditional love that Peter gives me in this breathwork session here in my father's apartment.*

Johanna's life and dreams illustrate the power of community and connection to heal grief. In her dream, there was a multigenerational party in her father's apartment to celebrate his life, and the practice of holotropic breathwork is designed to be done with the support of others. In her dream,

---

55. Note: The practice of holotropic breathwork is a therapeutic breathing practice. The guidelines of this practice specify not doing it alone; it generally involves three people: a trained guide, the breather, and a witness who monitors the breather for safety. For more information, see https://www.healthline.com/health/holotropic-breathwork.

Johanna engages with community practices designed for connection. We even see name sharing in this dream; the healer and her father share a name, adding yet another layer of interconnection.

Intergenerational Trauma Transmission, Loneliness, and the Healing Power of Attachment

In contrast to Johanna's story, there are many people who have not yet been able to access the healing of community and connection. Connection is one way we can help the body bear the burdens of past traumas. As I shared before, historical trauma can be passed down from generation to generation both epigenetically and via parenting styles. Repetitive traumas accumulate over time and deepen the wound. Through a combination of DNA, parenting, and societal norms, these responses can create habits, sensations, ideas, narratives, and beliefs. To be a good ancestor to your children and grandchildren, heal your body and soul from the wounds of the past to pass on healing and resilience, not wounding.

In recent years, researchers have learned about the ongoing effects of trauma from three newer branches of science: neuroscience, developmental psychopathology, and interpersonal neurobiology.[56] Neuroscience teaches us how the physical organ of the brain supports the mental processes of the mind, developmental psychopathology teaches us how adverse life experiences affect the developing mind and brain, and interpersonal neurobiology is the study of the interface between relationships and behaviors and how this affects biology and mindset. If your traumatic history (or your ancestors') includes abandonment, violence, gaslighting, chronic harsh criticism, or complicated loss, it can create ruptures and cause your relationships to suffer. Another trauma is loneliness.

Loneliness is not only an emotional or spiritual state, but also a physical state. The COVID-19 pandemic created an epidemic of loneliness as people were required to quarantine. Loneliness and a lack of connection do damage to the body as well as the soul. A lack of connection can be repaired in several ways, including attachment-focused therapeutic and somatic methods or interpersonal dreamwork in pairs and groups. Something shifts deep in

---

56. Van der Kolk, *The Body Keeps the Score*, 2.

the body and soul when we know we are not alone. Trauma can heal when we restore connection.

Accelerated Experiential Dynamic Psychotherapy (AEDP) is a therapeutic modality developed by Diana Fosha. It focuses on helping clients move through overwhelming emotional experiences while adding purposeful emotional engagement to help the brain embrace positive, adaptive change. With roots in the three branches of neuroscience, developmental psychopathology, and interpersonal neurobiology, AEDP seeks to undo the sense of aloneness that underpins most trauma. One of AEDP's primary tenants is that we are all hard-wired for healing, and with compassionate presence, we can all attain it. This makes a good case for doing your dreamwork and ancestral healing in the company of others. Whether it is with one other person or a group, the collective of caring will soothe your soul and facilitate the healing process. There is a saying in the business community: "Teamwork makes the dream work." In many ways, we can apply that motto to dreamwork as well.

EXERCISE
Sapphire Light Boundaries and Your Posse of Protection

This would be a useful exercise to do if you are exploring a nightmare or a disturbing dream. After you set clear boundaries, you are then better protected to go on to do the investigative and healing work.

1. Take a moment to surround yourself with a sapphire-blue container of light. Breathe it in for a count of three. As you breathe in, see this container of light becoming strong and bright. Breathe out any muddiness, darkness, or ickiness with a long exhale through the mouth.

2. As you sense the blue container of light around you, let this light protect you. Let it differentiate you from all other beings, all ancestors, all time, all space, and all dimensions. Let it clarify what is you and what is not you, what is now and what is not now. Let it be a clear boundary as well as a comfort.

3. Next, call on your posse of support. Perhaps they are with you in the room, or maybe they are simply in your mind's eye. Whether they are alive or dead, real or imaginary, human or angelic or magical or animal, let these beings surround you and accompany you on this journey. Allow yourself to be accompanied.

Neuroplasticity

Trauma produces cascades of neurochemicals in the body, such as adrenaline and cortisol, which create actual changes in the brain. These neurochemicals then in turn affect behaviors, relationships, and even physiology. The body's chemistry shows measurable changes in the cortisol, adrenal, and testosterone levels after exposure to a traumatic event.[57]

Researchers have spent years investigating methods that allow us to access the brain's innate neuroplasticity. Neuroplasticity is the brain's ability to adapt and change throughout life with new experiences, and to create the ability to strengthen new neural connections. This is in contrast to earlier theories that the brain was static and couldn't change much after childhood. You have the ability to change your brain's neural pathways, to break free of old, automatic cycles, and to create new habits that free you from the endless repetition of traumatic events. Daniel Siegel articulated the first two avenues for accessing neuroplasticity to make changes in life, and I added the third.[58]

1. **From the Top Down:** Talking, connecting, or reconnecting with others to gain a cognitive understanding of what you are experiencing, feeling, or dreaming about and why. These types of interventions primarily use the frontal lobe and pre-frontal cortex, also known as the thinking brain.

2. **From the Bottom Up:** Allowing the body to have the experiences it needs to soothe and support the system and somatically counteract the emotional residues of fear, rage, helplessness, or collapse that often accompany trauma. This includes a whole range of somatic

---
57. Yehuda and Lehrner, "Intergenerational Transmission of Trauma Effects."
58. Siegel, "Dr. Dan Siegel Explains 'Top Down' Constraints."

interventions, including yoga, Tai Chi, psychodrama, meditation, dance, music, art, energy-medicine based practices, and arts-based dreamwork.

3. **Medical Intervention:** The option of changing body chemistry to counteract excess (or lacking) neurochemicals that were affected by a traumatic event. Today, this includes psychiatric medications as well as the newer fields of ketamine-assisted psychotherapy and/or therapeutic use of psychedelics.

Slow Is the New Fast and the Window of Tolerance

Wounds and traumas may be personal, familial, ancestral, and/or cultural. To do this work, you need to go slowly and carefully to avoid retraumatizing your system. You need to develop a safe-enough space and a safe-enough relational space so you can let go, heal, and move on. The safe relational space is crucial—be accompanied this time. You don't have to do this alone. Your ancestors will appreciate the extra help too.

The window of tolerance is a concept developed by Daniel Siegel that proposes that everyone has a certain window within which they can comfortably experience, process, and integrate difficult experiences. If an individual goes above or below their window of tolerance, they enter states of hyperarousal (fight or flight) or hypoarousal (freeze). In hyper- and hypoarousal, the thinking brain is overtaken by the emotion brain. When you are in danger or outside your window of tolerance, you react instead of respond; you cannot incorporate the skills of your thinking brain.

"Staying inside your window" is a phrase I often use when working with nightmares or trauma to avoid retraumatization. You can work to the edges of your window, but not beyond. Feeling uncomfortable is okay; feeling unsafe is not. If you feel you have gone above or below your window, that's a sign to back off, slow down, and recenter.

The Embodied Nature

```
┌─────────────────────────────────────────┐
│            Hyperarousal                 │
│  high energy, anxiety, anger, overwhelm │
│   hypervigilance, flight/fight, chaotic │
└─────────────────────────────────────────┘

        Window of Tolerance
     ∿∿∿∿∿∿∿∿∿∿∿∿∿∿∿
   grounded, flexible, open/curious, present,
         able to emotionally self-regulate
                                              Hormonal
┌─────────────────────────────────────────┐   activity
│            Hypoarousal                  │
│   shut down, numb, depression, passive, │
│     withdrawn, freeze, shame            │
└─────────────────────────────────────────┘

──────────────────────────────────►
                Time
```

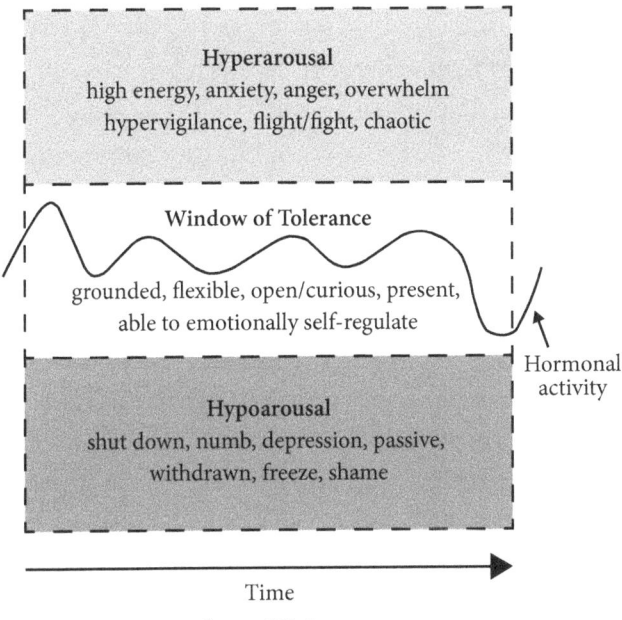

Window of Tolerance

When you are inside your window of tolerance, you can approach nightmares, trauma, or the struggles and pain of the ancestors with your thinking brain, not just your emotion brain. In your window, you can cope with challenges, handle stress, and remain regulated. The goal is to widen or broaden your window of tolerance as much as you can. If you are a trauma survivor, you may feel unsafe in your own body, in relationships with others, and in the world at large. Learning how to enlarge your window of tolerance can help you access a felt sense of safety more quickly. A wider window also expands your resilience when doing dreamwork with hurt ancestors. There are several techniques for stress management and staying centered that can help you stay inside your window so you can be a resource for yourself and your loved ones.[59]

---

59. See "How to Help Your Clients Understand Their Window of Tolerance."

EXERCISE
Grounding in the Present and Attaching

1. Take a moment and breathe. Put your feet on the ground and settle into your body. Whether you are in a room or in nature, notice your surroundings. Connect yourself with the here and now.

2. Notice the nicest thing in the surrounding area and name it. For example, "that flowering tree in front of me," "my cat," or "my wedding ring." Access this touchstone a few times, then close or lower your eyes. Use this touchstone to return to a feeling of calm if you become upset at any point during this exercise. It is an associational cue for the present.

3. Next, identify a bad dream or nightmare that had to do with your ancestors. Think about the dream for just a moment, then move away from it—don't linger right now. Then, notice your internal felt sense. Do you feel anxiety, fear, or sadness? Where do you feel it in your body?

4. Now, invite someone into your space with whom you feel close, beloved, connected, and seen. Spiritual, human, and animal beings are all invited! Sense them beside you. Feel their presence.

5. Now, gently return to that bad dream or nightmare again, and notice what is different. Let yourself toggle back and forth between your supportive connection and the dream. Notice the difference in your felt sense in your body. Chances are, even though the nightmare is still there, you feel less frightened and accompanied in your journey.

The Power of Choice

Once you have identified and differentiated what trauma you are carrying from your own life versus what trauma you inherited, you are then gifted with the power of choice. Choice is a direct opposite of the original state a person was in when experiencing a trauma: being/feeling trapped, helpless, or powerless.

When you feel that you have no choice, your body and nervous system perceive that as a threat. The work now is to discern if the threat is still true for you currently. What was then, and what is now? Is there a difference? To heal, you need strong, clear boundaries between the past, the present, and the future, even as you travel between them. You also need strong boundaries between yourself and others, even as you connect with them.

What Are You Carrying?

You carry the epigenetic and genetic imprints of those who came before you, but you also have a choice. You do not need to continue to carry what is not your own baggage. Ask yourself, *Is this mine to hold or carry?* If the answer is no, are you able to simply put the baggage down or let it go once you have identified this, or is there some healing work you need to do with your ancestors first?

Embedded in much of the works of Holocaust survivor and author Elie Wiesel is the concept that people become the stories they hear and the stories they tell. As you identify what you are carrying, you have the potential to then change the stories you tell yourself. Marion, my first consultant out of grad school, taught me the phrase "I am the story I tell myself I am." That wisdom has stayed with me as I continue to work to stay aware of the unconscious stories I tell myself so that I have the gifts of choice and change.

Muscle Memory

I remember when I learned how to ride a bike. I started with a tricycle, balancing first on three solid wheels, then graduated to a two-wheeler with training wheels. Then the training wheels came off and an adult ran behind me with one hand on the seat until suddenly, magically, I was riding on my own! I might have taken a few spills in the beginning, but after a while, I just hopped on the bike and rode without having to think about it at all. No matter how long it has been since I rode a bike, I can still hop on and ride because my body remembers how. I developed muscle memory that simply takes over without any cognition needed on my part.

I currently am having an interesting experience with muscle memory. Years ago, when I was in my twenties, I had a horseback riding accident and was thrown from a galloping horse. I landed on my coccyx, but I did not break any bones. A few months ago, several of my friends asked me why I was limping. It wasn't a limp from an injury, but my misaligned hips were catching up with me. I was aware of it too; I felt like a duck with a kind of waddle.

My trainer is also an expert in sports rehab. He did an assessment, concurred with the diagnosis of "uneven pelvis," and supervised me as I did some exercises to even things out. To my delight, after just one week I had made some real progress in rebalancing. Here's where the catch comes in: After decades of being uneven, my body had acclimated to that state of being. In its newly balanced state, it protested mightily. The next week, I began having aches and pains in hitherto non-problematic body parts! My team of bodyworkers (chiropractor, acupuncturist, trainer) agreed that my body was realigning itself in response to my newly balanced hips, and it would just take time for things to sort themselves out.

On further reflection, I remembered that my mom also had a limp later in life, enough so that my siblings and I encouraged her to get it looked at. She had an imbalance in her hip and had that same waddle I was experiencing. We never figured out why this limp showed up for my mom. Was it structural, an inherited body type, or from an accident during childhood? Or was it inherited in some way from her own mother's life? There may be something there. I was not able to find out more information since my mother died several years ago, but it did make me wonder: Was this imbalance inherited in some way beyond a fall from a horse? In my bone-knowing, it feels like there is truth there. Now, my sports rehab work helps me feel connected to my mom. I am choosing to embrace the intention that my work will help balance out anything that my mom may still be carrying on the other side, and that this will go as far back in my family line as necessary for healing.

You can have the equivalent of muscle memory in ancestral lineage and in your dreams. One of my favorite examples is using the body's muscle memory to retrieve a lost dream. Many of us have had the experience of waking up and going about our morning routine only to suddenly realize we had a dream that we can't remember. Next time this happens to you, take a moment to lie back down in bed in the same position you slept in. If you were sleeping on your left side with your hands folded under your chin and your knees bent, do that. If you are a stomach sleeper and had your face turned to the right, do that. Hold still in that position for a few moments. Nine times out of ten, the dream will reappear to you. Muscle memory saves the day! I never cease to be amazed at how well this works. This time, write down the details of your dream right away to honor the process.

Bodily Concepts of Neuroception and Interoception

One of the reasons I made progress with my unbalanced pelvis fairly quickly is that I have been practicing the arts of focusing and interoception for some years. I could focus my mind on the body part being worked with, engaging it more easily than someone who hasn't had the practice. Interoception is the ability to be aware of internal sensations in the body, including the rate of your heart, being hungry, and being hot or cold. It has also been called *multisensory integration*, which includes body noticing and body listening. Once we notice, we can listen, and once we listen, we can engage and differentiate. So, when my trainer asked me to put my attention on engaging specific muscles in my body, I could access the right muscle groups. For example, when I was asked to engage my glutes rather than my quads to do a bridge pose, I could differentiate between them once I put my mindful attention on them. Think of interoception as putting your mind on or in your body. Once practiced, you will get the "Oh, there it is!" feeling more and more easily.

Cultivating your own interoception capabilities will help you more quickly identify when something is out of balance in your system. As you make the connections between your bodily sensations and your emotional state, you can use that awareness to address these feelings. When my daughter was young, she hadn't yet learned to identify her internal signals of hunger and could get grumpy and irritable because she needed some food in her belly (a common phenomenon in children—and some adults as well). Cuing her to identify the physical and accompanying emotional states of needing a meal or a snack made her life (and mine) much easier. Nowadays, there is a word for this: *hangry*, a mash-up of *hungry* and *angry*, short for "Do you think that you are irritable because you need to eat something?"

Similar to interoception is the concept of neuroception. *Neuroception*, a phrase coined by Stephen Porges, is how our internal autonomous neurocircuits decide (without engaging our thinking brain) if a situation is safe, dangerous, or threatening. In intergenerational transmitted trauma, epigenetic neurocircuitry is still resonating with events that happened long ago, to parents, grandparents, or beyond. Input from an individual's current surroundings is overridden by the input from their internal inherited world, which is telling them they are still being abandoned, persecuted, or starved. This inner circuitry gets stuck on replay, as it cannot differentiate between then and now.

Neuroception listens to three streams of input:

1. Input inside the body
2. Input outside the body, via the environment
3. The resonance between the internal nervous system and the external system, which includes the environment and the people around you

Humans are more porous than we realize, and children are especially so. Before they learn how to verbally communicate, everything is absorbed through the body as somatosensory information. Infants and small children feel things in their bodies without the mitigating bridge of communication to provide some cognitive distancing. As adults, we have the gift of language to provide a bridge of self-awareness to what were only undifferentiated feelings before we had the ability to form thoughts via language.

Co-regulation, the ability to help to calm, heal, and regulate each other while in relationship, is key to this way of working. This is why healing yourself and your ancestors so often needs to be done in connection with others who can help with co-regulation. Parents and caregivers were your first co-regulators, and if they were not sufficient—or if the trauma they experienced affected their capacity to lend emotional, physical, and energetic support—then later in life, your partners, friends, and therapeutic caregivers can assist in this development.

When you work with others in a dream circle, the resonance of co-regulation passes around the group and can accentuate the healing process. Both in the here and now, and in the then and there, awareness and connection heal.

You can practice this in your waking work and in your dreams. As the beginning of this chapter highlighted, when you do dreamwork, you can ask yourself and others, "Where do you feel that in your body? And what is the sensation there?" Then, the group can notice it with you as well and provide feedback to your dream from their responses to it.

Embodied Memory Traces

The heavy weight of ancestral pain can be carried as a physical burden in subsequent generations. It can harden—calcify, if you will—from emotional or spiritual pain into physical symptoms and illness if the source is not addressed. This is part of the premise of psychosomatic pain. Psychosomatic pain is real, but Western medicine has not found a physiological cause for this hurt. Re-establishing the ownership of your body is a crucial step toward healing. Repair may be needed at many levels of being.

A friend of mine suffers from terrible migraine headaches, usually feeling them the worst on the front right side of her head. They have been debilitating at times, interfering with her work and her life, and she has been chasing down treatment options for years. In one conversation, we were talking about her family of origin and her brother's suicide in his late teens. I suddenly remembered that she had told me he died from a gunshot wound. When I asked her if I remembered correctly, she responded, "Yes, he shot himself in the head."

I asked, "Where on his head?"

"On the right front side of his forehead." She paused. "Oh."

She had the aha moment of knowing that this was connected. Her next steps were to heal from the trauma of her brother's suicide on a bodily level in addition to the work she had already done on the cognitive and emotional levels.

Marisa's Story

A client of mine, Marisa, suffered from chronic fatigue syndrome for years. This somewhat mysterious but very real illness is often hard to diagnose and does not have a clear path to treatment. It is characterized by exhaustion; muscle aches and pains; brain fog; extreme sensitivity to external stimuli, such as loud noise or bright lights; and, not surprisingly, mood fluctuations. Marisa said there were times in her life when she frequently had "three-bath days" because nothing brought any relief to her achy muscles and the sense of pressure on her chest except for a warm bathtub.

In therapy, we focused on helping Marisa cope with this condition as well as paying attention to her dreams. One day, she said, "I don't know why, but I keep having dreams that I am buried alive. I can feel the weight of the dirt piled up on me in my dream, sort of like the achiness I feel in my joints and muscles."

As we followed the threads of the dreamscape, Marisa recalled that in her dream, she was accused of being a witch in a former life, and her punishment was having layers of earth piled on her to see if she could use magic to free herself. She couldn't, and in that lifetime, she died from this test. After recounting the dream, Marisa said that it felt like a past-life experience that she was reliving now.

It may be hard to discern between a past-life experience and an ancestral memory. If you can't trace the dream's themes to a known ancestor, or an experience that would have been likely for an ancestor, then the source of the dream images and experiences may come from somewhere else, possibly a past life. What happens to the soul after the body dies is something that we don't know for certain, and past lives may or may not be part of your belief system. Did Marisa really have a past-life experience like this? We can't know for sure, but the symptoms she was experiencing in day-to-day life were eerily consistent with what it might have felt like to be buried under layers of earth. So, Marisa and I decided to work with this dream as we might work with a dream memory of ancestral lineage. We wanted to try to find a way to bring some sort of healing or closure to the experience so that it didn't continue to follow her around in this and subsequent lifetimes. The bottom line is that something was disturbing her body and soul, so we took it seriously to work toward healing and resolution.

Marisa realized during our dreamwork that she couldn't simply undo the trauma of being buried alive, as it had happened to her witch-woman self. In Tapas Acupressure Technique (TAT), a meridian-based mind/body therapeutic method, one of the steps is to say, "It happened, and it's over now, and I can relax and heal and move on." Marisa and I used that framework to process her dream: It happened as Marisa dreamed it, but she recognized that she could still free the soul of this entombed woman. So, with beautiful clarity, she connected across time and space to a barely marked grave in Salem, MA, and gave recognition to the soul that was trapped there. With her encouragement, and with an entourage of helpful angels she had invited in, Marisa guided that soul to rise out of the ground it was trapped in, relieving the pressure of the dirt so it could join in the light and freedom of the afterlife. When we were done, Marisa said she felt a sense of peacefulness course through her being.

As we continued to work together over the following weeks and months, Marisa found that she was less and less achy and did not experience a single three-bath day. As her body felt stronger and less fatigued, she could support that shift with gentle exercise that further strengthened her sense of well-being. She had the energy and vitality to spend time with her grandchildren as well as to get back to her writing.

The Ancestor Syndrome

In addition to the neuroanatomy of epigenetic inheritance, there is a transgenerational psychotherapy concept called *ancestor syndrome*.[60] It seems that the unconscious has a good memory! Ancestor syndrome may be showing up when you act or react to something unseen, feel sad for no apparent reason, or feel irritable for no reason. Usually, these states last for days or weeks. You may even have dreams that reflect your emotional state. One day, you'll notice or remember that it is the anniversary of a significant event in your family, such as your mother's death or your deceased father's birthday. Suddenly, your dreams and emotional state makes sense in this context, and this is often accompanied by a flush of relief as the unknown becomes known.

If you go back several generations, you will likely notice repetitions of family accidents, marriages, births, deaths, etc. at the same age. For example, my friend Sue's mom got cancer at age forty-eight, and so did Sue. My

---

60. See Schützenberger's *The Ancestor Syndrome* to learn more.

colleague Marlene's mom had her first child at thirty-six, and so did Marlene. Clients and friends often tell me they were exquisitely conscious of the age their parent died and breathed a sigh of relief when they passed that age marker. Both my brothers and I breathed a sigh of relief when we passed the age of forty-nine, as that was the age our father died. Dodged the family bullet, as it were. Can you resonate with this, especially if you had a parent who died relatively young?

Paying attention to your genogram and your family history as well as your dreams can help you identify times of the year that have meaning for you. This can alert you to the potential need to honor your forebears, care for yourself, and be clear about what is yours and what is theirs. The susceptibility to repetition seems to become diluted over generations, particularly if you have made the past visible and done your healing work.

What Happens When Grieving Is Unfinished or Never Begun?

Ungrieved sorrows or losses never get metabolized by the body. Instead, they sit and turn sour or rotten at the core of your being and are at risk of metastasizing both emotionally and physically. If you have lost someone and survived trauma yourself, you need to make meaning out of your survival and honor the memories of those you lost so that you don't continue to carry this in your gut, head, or heart. Every survivor carries the pain of their experiences, and survivor's guilt is a real thing. If not acknowledged, addressed, and grieved, the next generation then inherits your unmetabolized loss—and the responsibility of doing something with the loss or grief they had no part in creating. This is an enormous responsibility.

Unmetabolized losses demand to be heard and acknowledged. You may dream of ancestors who are still in pain, who need healing and resolution, and/or who are stuck in their anger and resentment. These are often ancestors who shout rather than whisper. Not seeking revenge against others takes a great deal of courage and fortitude. When ancestors come through in your dreams or in waking encounters with pain or grudges that they want you to continue acting out, you need alternatives to heal this legacy and keep it from continuing forward.

The Embodied Nature

Trauma, Hormonal Effects, and Polyvagal Theory

When confronted with extreme stress, the body initiates many chemical reactions to facilitate a quick escape. The amygdala, located in the limbic system, is the region of the brain that alerts the body to danger and activates hormonal systems. When the hormones noradrenaline and adrenaline are activated, the results are quickened breathing, a faster pulse, and an increased release of energy. This energy can help people run away from the perceived danger faster, or it can engage a response that requires coping with the stressor head-on. Once the immediate danger has passed, other hormones (particularly cortisol) help terminate stress-activated reactions.

When this automatic process is not completed, individuals get stuck on replay. The system doesn't rebalance itself. This contributes to the development of PTSD. Studies have shown that trauma survivors with PTSD have higher levels of noradrenaline and lower levels of cortisol.[61] The body keeps the score, indeed, even at the level of cortisol production and sensitivity. If knowledge is power, then the more we learn about this phenomenon, the more effectively we can prevent and treat PTSD. If we can better understand PTSD, we may be able to prevent its transmission across generational lines.

Polyvagal Theory

Stephen Porges originated the research on polyvagal theory. It further explains the mind/body connection and how we react to stimuli through the body without the benefit of the thinking mind. The vagus nerve touches almost every part of the body, running from the brainstem to the lungs, heart, and all digestive organs. The word *vagus* comes from New Latin and means "wandering," an apt term for this nerve that wanders throughout the whole body.[62] One place the vagus nerve does not connect to is the thinking brain, the cortex. It only connects at the brain level to the brainstem, which is affectionately referred to as the "lizard brain."

---

61. Yehuda et al., "Holocaust Exposure Induced Intergenerational Effects on FKBP5 Methylation."
62. *Merriam-Webster Dictionary*, "vagus," accessed February 25, 2025, https://www.merriam-webster.com/dictionary/vagus.

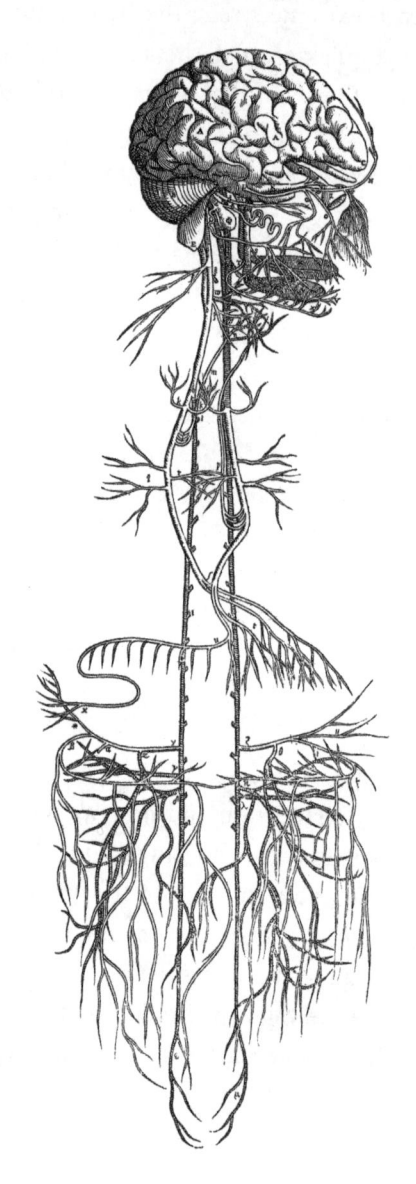

Vagus Nerve

The Embodied Nature

To emphasize, the one part of the brain that the vagus nerve doesn't connect to is the thinking cortex. Therefore, when a person is triggered into a trauma response—whatever the source of the original trauma—they don't have access to their thinking brain to help them differentiate between what is in their current environment and what is in the past. They cannot mediate what they feel in their body. This is a crucial piece of information and underlies why people cannot solely rely on their ability to think their way out of a situation.

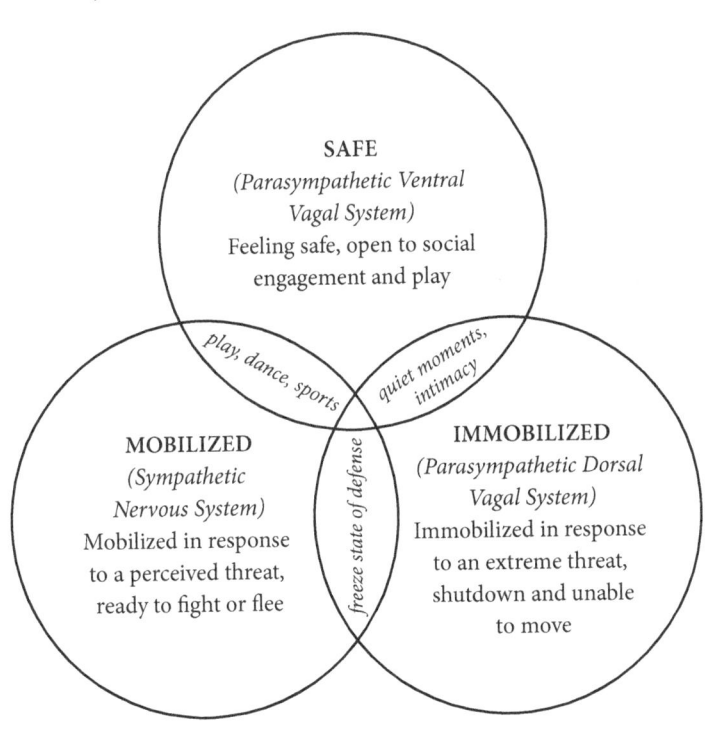

SAFE
(Parasympathetic Ventral Vagal System)
Feeling safe, open to social engagement and play

play, dance, sports — *quiet moments, intimacy*

MOBILIZED
(Sympathetic Nervous System)
Mobilized in response to a perceived threat, ready to fight or flee

freeze state of defense

IMMOBILIZED
(Parasympathetic Dorsal Vagal System)
Immobilized in response to an extreme threat, shutdown and unable to move

Three Polyvagal States

The nervous system is a complex network or nerves and neuronal cells that transmit messages to and from the brain and spinal cord to all parts of the body, enabling us to move, think, perceive, and react to the world. Above is a graphic that illustrates the three states your nervous system may rest in.

The urge to fight, flee, or freeze are common responses to traumatic circumstances. These classic responses are often necessary to survive an assault: You get away as quickly as possible, you fight back, or you shut down in a collapsed state that freezes emotion until it is safe to feel again. The key is to know when you can move out of the triggered trauma response and move into what is called the ventral vagal state of calm, safe presence.

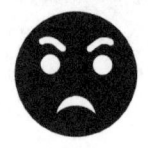

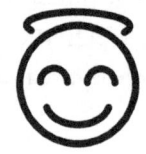

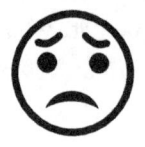

Three-Emotion Polyvagal Theory

Body-Centered Healing

If we can inherit trauma, we can inherent resilience. My friend Daphne recently learned that her skill as a seamstress and clothing designer may have been inherited from her maternal grandfather. Recently, Daphne reached out to some far-flung cousins to make family connections. In the process, she learned that her grandfather was a skilled tailor and created clothing for several stores and "persons of note" after coming to America from Italy. While clothing design is not what I usually think of when I think of inherited ancestral gifts, it certainly is a gift! Daphne's grandfather used this skill to get back on his feet after an arduous immigration experience in the early nineteenth century, and Daphne used this skill to get back on her feet after a series of health crises that left her unable to continue her previous work.

You can turn to your waking and sleeping dreams for source material and messages. When you can learn to settle in your body, you can more deeply relax, which can lead to restorative sleep and informative dreams. If you work with others, your ability to settle in your body can help your client, friend, or family member settle as well. The space between you becomes part of the healing matrix. This ability is related to mirror neurons.

Mirror neurons are specific neurons in the brain that react when we execute a certain act and when we witness someone else execute that act or a similar one. They facilitate learning and may be the neural basis for empathy. For example, if you see someone yawn, you may yawn. If someone laughs, you may laugh. With the help of mirror neurons, you can

The Embodied Nature

access resources that you couldn't access on your own when you are not grounded in the present.

Menakem tells us that this ability to settle is often a prelude to deeper healing.[63] Since the response to danger must be first to escape or survive, slowing it all down once the actual danger has passed is a pathway to healing. You may need to rest and protect before you can slow down. That is okay too; listen to your body's messages closely.

The ability to bounce back, to adapt, and to be flexible are key traits in moving from PTSD to PTSG: Post Trauma Spiritual Growth, an expression I coined in my book *PTSDreams*. As you practice somatic flexibility in your body and your dreamwork, you can pass the ability to heal and move on to your ancestors and descendants as well. You can learn resilience; it is not a trait that is only inherited. Resiliency allows you to believe in yourself and in your ability to make changes in life.

EXERCISE
"I Feel, I Am"

You can practice sitting with your discomfort, whether from a dream or everyday life, and remind yourself that this discomfort was originally intended to be protective, not defective. Try this exercise when you are in a safe location.

1. Recall a moment when you felt triggered or had a larger-than-life response to a stimulus. For example, did you jump out of your skin when you heard a car backfire and feel panic? The anxiety might not have subsided even after you identified the source of the upset. Find your own example.

2. Identify the emotion the triggering moment brings up in you.

3. Notice that right now, in this moment, you are safe. Then, sit with the sensation and the emotion for a moment. Notice the discomfort. Breathe into it. Name it. For example, "I feel anxious, and my chest is tight." You could also

---
63. Menakem, *My Grandmother's Hands*.

say, "My chest feels tight and uncomfortable. Thank you for alerting me to danger when I needed it before."

4. When you feel ready, say out loud, "I feel uncomfortable and anxious right now, but I am safe."

5. Practice diaphragmatic breathing: belly extending with the in breath, belly contracting with the out breath. Continue to do this until your breathing has become regular. You may notice that the upset has passed.

This is a variation on a mind/body exercise called, appropriately enough, "I feel, I am." First, you accept the discomfort. Then, you sit with it. Finally, you allow it to move through you. Embodied dreamwork practices are ideal for this, as are contemplative practices such as yoga and meditation.

Shaking It Off

Peter Levine, the creator of the mind/body healing modality somatic experiencing, studied animals in the wild to learn why animals didn't seem to develop PTSD, even though they live in the world of predator and prey all the time. Levine observed that following a successful escape from a predator (utilizing the fight, flight, freeze, or play dead responses), animals exhibited a distinct movement pattern.[64] Almost without exception, once they ascertained they were safe, the animal performed some version of shaking it off. For example, once a rabbit has outrun a fox, it will shake itself or ripple the skin on its back to discharge the energy of adrenaline. Birds ruffle their feathers. Deer twitch. Other animals roll, jump, or run in short circles. Once excess adrenaline has been discharged, the animal returns to its normal lifestyle. Levine describes this renegotiation of the initial stuck/frozen response as completing the incomplete mobility that sets in during a freeze response. Finishing the movement to safety that could not be completed at the time of the event itself allows the body to complete the repair that was interrupted.[65]

---

64. Levine and Frederick, *Waking the Tiger*, 97–98.
65. Levine and Frederick, *Waking the Tiger*, 99–123.

The Embodied Nature

Physical discharge of some sort is a crucial part of moving through trauma. It is safe to assume that the majority of your ancestors were not aware of the biological need to clear the embodied effects of their distress. Others may not have had a chance to do so if they were on the move, looking for safety, or if they were struggling to support their families even when the immediate danger had passed. Today, many people remain unaware of this biological need. However, now that you know, you can incorporate this protective discharge of tension when tuning in to your ancestors' suffering or after a nightmare or traumatic experience of your own.

> **EXERCISE**
> *Shaking It Off*
> Use this exercise after you have had an upsetting dream.
>
> 1. First, write or record details of your dream. It is important to solidify the memory of the images and feelings before moving forward. You can then work with the dream in more depth later if you have anchored the details concretely.
> 2. Now, see if you can simply allow your body to move through its automatic somatic responses. Give yourself permission to shake, quiver, or tremble.
> 3. If you can sit with these uncomfortable somatic responses and let them run their course, they will resolve into feelings of warmth, relaxation, and calm. Then, you will be able to get up and go about your day, much as the gazelle grazes after the tiger has gone.

Gwen's Story

Sometimes when you are lucky, or when you have been working with your dreams and your body for some time, you will get a form of release right within your dream.

Gwen was born seven years after the Holocaust ended, and while some of her family members escaped, some did not and were murdered. Growing up in a safe, healthy environment, one lens through which Gwen sees her life is as a resting one: a time of reprieve and repair from the horrors and trauma her ancestors experienced. She also recognizes the impacts that remain, as her own fear of basements and dark places may be a reflection of her familial legacy.

Gwen had been working on her dream healing in one of my dream groups for about fifteen years when she had this dream.

> I am dancing with cymbals on my fingers, like castanets. It is a spiral, snaky kind of dance.

In group, we asked questions and offered thoughts about the meaning of this dream, using the respectful format "If this were my dream, I'd wonder about..." Gwen told us that this was a happy dream, as she enjoyed making music. She plays the piano and violin. We noticed that in this dream, the tips of Gwen's fingers were making music, not being bitten down in anxiety as they were in waking life. Someone in the group tuned in to the wonderful pun of cymbal/symbol, and we explored the symbol of the finger cymbals. Gwen's Hebrew name is Miriam, and in the Tanach (Hebrew Bible), Miriam led the people in song and dance with her tambourine after the Exodus from slavery in Egypt.[66] For Gwen, the tambourine was a symbol of hope and release, as were the cymbals. The final layer of this short but powerful dream was the spiral, snaky dance. The snake sheds its skin to be reborn anew, and the ouroboros eats its own tail in an unending cycle of renewal.

In this dream, Gwen is both dancing and making music by moving the cymbals rhythmically with her fingers. In this way, Gwen is exploring two forms of movement. So, when you think about embodied healing, this dream contains several elements. You can use this as inspiration for your own embodied dream healing by utilizing music and dance to heal pain and invite joy.

Body-Centered Dreamwork Practices

There are several body-oriented practices that can aid in healing nightmares, bad dreams, and ancestral legacies. I will explicate some of them

---

66. Exodus 15:20–21.

more fully in the coming chapters, but for now, start with body befriending as a key concept.

Many modern healing practices speak of the body as our greatest teacher. As you befriend the body you live in, you can address current body-based struggles such as feeling safe inside your own body, poor body image, inherited sensitivities, and trauma responses. (If you are struggling with these, please consider working with a therapist to help you pace yourself and remain safe.) You can also honor and appreciate the ways you already live at peace with yourself inside your body. Some of these struggles and acceptances are yours, from your own personal life experiences, and others are part of your intergenerational inheritance, for better or for worse.

Many bad dreams involve danger or threat to the physical body. While your departed ancestors are no longer embodied, they were when they experienced their pain and traumas, so if you work with your dreams in an embodied fashion and move toward befriending and accepting the body you have, you can send these healing messages back to your ancestors as well. Linear time is an illusion, especially in the dreamscape, while lucid dreaming, or while doing dreamwork in waking life.

Dual awareness is another element of body-based healing. It can help you cultivate the ability to be in the past and the present simultaneously. Thus, it allows you to remain centered and grounded in current reality while attending to the other times and places in your life or the lives of your ancestors that still need healing. Start with safety first. Always. Remind yourself that you are safe in the here and now. As you practice ancestral dreamwork, remember to utilize the exercises I've already shared, such as "Grounding in the Present and Attaching." These include others with appropriate levels of accompaniment and/or guidance to help you stay safe and oriented.

The following list identifies several body-oriented dreamwork methods, including some described in this chapter and additional methods that you can explore.

- **Cultivating Interoception:** The ability to put your mind on or in your body to be consciously aware of it (from polyvagal theory).

- **Focusing:** Cultivating a felt sense and allowing yourself to track and follow it (based on the work of Eugene Gendlin).
- **Empowerment Postures:** Physically creating postural changes that bring you and your dream body into greater alignment. These can shift negative emotional states to positive emotional states through somatic experiencing work, or variations on the "superhero" pose of legs firmly planted, hands on hips, chest up, and head lifted.
- **Psychodrama/Constellation Work:** Physical reenactment of dream scenes or family dynamics in a group setting (based on Hellinger's work and aspects of Internal Family Systems).
- **Somatic Experiencing/Psychomotor Psychotherapy:** Designed by Peter Levine and Pat Ogden respectively, both methods attend to the physicality of emotional states and offer integrated techniques.
- **Yoga:** Can include meditation, breathwork, and body postures/movements.
- **Breathwork:** A wide variety of breathing styles that can help calm the nervous system and settle the body to be better able to gently approach nightmares and ancestral healing work.
- **Mind/Body Energy Methods:** Integrated mind/body therapeutic techniques that can be learned initially from a trained practitioner, then adapted or used on your own as self-help techniques. Includes EMDR (Eye Movement Desensitization and Reprocessing), TAT (Tapas Acupressure Technique), and EFT (Emotional Freedom Technique).

* * *

Trauma is something that initially involves the body and human instinct. After that, its effects spread to the mind and spirit. Engaging the body can help you uncouple the fear that accompanied the trauma. Feel free to add sound (sighs, grunts, shouts, or whispers) along with your movements to release the fear response. In this way, you will find your voice and give voice to those who were silenced.

There is a prayer that contains this message: "All the world is just a narrow bridge, and our main task is not to make ourselves afraid." Let us now move to a structured method of dreamwork that was based on effective trauma treatment and created specifically for nightmare healing.

SEVEN

GAIA METHOD APPLIED TO ANCESTRAL DREAMS AND NIGHTMARES

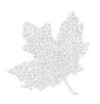

> One of the great gifts of darkness and
> the night is our capacity to dream.
> —**Estelle Frankel,** *The Wisdom of Not Knowing*

In chapter 1, I identified six types of contact you may have with your visiting ancestors. You may hear or feel these calls through your dreams; in your waking life, via dreamish states; or through the epigenetic inheritances and storylines in your body, mind, and soul.

1. "I am still here, and you are not alone."
2. "Take these gifts, blessings, or apologies."
3. "Let me help, heal, or warn you."
4. "Please, please help and heal me; I am still suffering."
5. "Watch out: This old grudge has not yet been resolved."
6. "Carry on my name and gifts to your children and your children's children. Remember."

The first three are usually warm, pleasant, or healing calls: *I'm still with you, I can bless you,* and *I want to offer you help, advice, or healing.* When your ancestors whisper or call in these ways, it is easier to connect with them, and you are likely delighted and appreciative of their call.

The final call to remember them and to tell their story can take more time and processing on your part, particularly if your ancestor's story was suppressed or kept secret. But once you have connected with their legacy and committed to keeping it alive for future generations to learn from, you usually don't need special protections or guides to allow you to retell their story and honor them concretely in life.

However, when calls four or five come through, be it in a shout or a whisper, your task is more difficult. You may not know what to do, how to respond, how to help, or how to keep yourself from feeling overwhelmed. You may feel anxious or unprepared for these kinds of contacts and requests. I created the GAIA method as a protective scaffolding for nightmare healing when the pain of contact is more than a person can bear to work with.

GAIA stands for Guided Active Imagination Approach. This two-pronged dreamwork method offers the scaffolding and support needed to be able to deal with nightmares from a place of calmness and curiosity rather than fear and overwhelm. First described in my book *Modern Dreamwork* and expanded upon in my second book, *PTSDreams*, I will now teach you how to use and apply this method when working with ancestral dreams *and* nightmares. Using this approach will help you stay safe, grounded, and accompanied while doing this work. Then, you will be able to enter the world of your ancestors to put an end to their grudges or heal their unsoothed pain.

I am reminded of an old therapist joke (you have to be able to laugh at yourself in this profession): A traveler shows up at the airport for their flight and is directed to check in at a luggage counter called Emotional Baggage Check-In. They are asked by the attendant, "Has your baggage been with you at all times?" to which the traveler replies, "Unfortunately, yes." The attendant then asks, "Did anyone ask you to carry anything for them?" to which the traveler replies, "You have no idea how many times!"

Because trauma interferes with a person's ability to be safe, to feel safe, and to create safety both during and after a traumatic event, the creation of a safe-enough environment in which to do healing work is the first priority. You need to go gently, with supports and resources. Overzealous attempts to move into the belly of the nightmare too quickly can result in retraumatization. Treading carefully as you enter and exit this territory allows you to avoid the extremes of getting too overwhelmed or becoming dissociated. In order to build sufficient resilience to process emotional residue, it is better to start building safety slowly and surely. In other words, build the ground floor and the scaffolding before scaling the walls. The key phrase "S and S" can guide you: safety and support.

Foundational Pillars of the GAIA Method

The GAIA method rests on two foundational pillars: those of current, best-practice trauma treatment, and those of the Jungian principles of active imagination.

Best-Practice Trauma Treatment

Trauma scholar Dr. Judith Herman outlined a protocol of three phases of healing from trauma back in the 1980s, and these guidelines hold true today. The three phases she articulated are:

1. Establishing safety and stabilization

2. Remembrance and mourning (which includes telling the story of the traumatic event)

3. Reconnection and integration[67]

These are not meant to be strictly linear stages, for trauma treatment (as well as grief work and dreamwork) does not follow a neat, linear path. Rather, the stages are to be revisited and reinforced in a spiraling Möbius strip as needed, as new material emerges and new challenges occur. The establishment of safety, addressed in stage one, needs to be periodically revisited in the face of new information or new stressors in therapy, in dreamwork, and in life. Safety includes having the ability to tolerate, regulate, and manage strong emotions that show up in waking and dreaming life.

Herman's phases are redescribed here with attention to their applicability to our work on intergenerational trauma transmission.

Stage One: Developing the resources needed to be able to handle the nightmares, memories, and emotions associated with intergenerational trauma. Herman's safety and stabilization imply developing skills and resources to calm the body and mind, to stay centered

---

67. Herman, *Trauma and Recovery*, 155.

and focused, and to be accompanied by whomever or whatever you need to face your unsettling dreams or anxious ancestors.

Stage Two: Working with your resources through a variety of integrated mind/body/spirit practices and dreamwork methods to discern what is needed for each ancestral download. Name what has been held in silence or secret and process what has not yet been processed. For our purposes, Herman's remembrance and mourning may mean facing, unraveling, revealing, and allowing grief to take place.

Stage Three: Releasing, returning, healing, letting go, and moving on with the wholeness of your own being. In other words, carrying only what is yours. Self-integration here is recognizing who you are and who you aren't, honoring those who came before you while still having intact boundaries. This step in Herman's formulation often involves a reconnection with community and an action step of giving back in some way. This is the action and meaning-making step of dreamwork.

As Viktor Frankl writes in *Man's Search for Meaning*, between the stimulus and the response there is space, and in that space in between, we have the power of choice—the power to choose our own attitude in any given situation. You have the freedom to change yourself and how you hold any given situation. Meaning making then becomes part of your personal growth and spiritual path. Honoring the paths of your ancestors and the trials they suffered and then doing something concrete, however large or small, makes meaning out of their experiences. So does sharing their stories with your descendants so that you may all live the phrase "never forget" and hopefully prevent these traumas form reoccurring.

Active Imagination

Active imagination is one of the foundations of Jungian dreamwork practice. It can be defined as dropping down into the landscape of the dream in waking life to create the ability to interact with the dream and the characters therein.

GAIA Method Applied to Ancestral Dreams and Nightmares

Active imagination is a tool for transformation. You can use it to freely imagine the thoughts, feelings, and alternative actions that your dream characters may take. Once you have established enough safety, if you meet a ghost or a murderer in a dream during your active imagination processing, you will then be able to talk to the dream characters and hear their answers.

In utilizing active imagination, you maintain connections with both your waking consciousness and with your dream characters. Add the active transformational possibilities that emerge when you combine these two states of consciousness to create a third option or form.

It can be challenging to do active imagination work on your own, since you are looking at the back of your own head, so to speak—that is hard to do without someone who can help hold the mirror! It is not impossible, though, and if you would like to try active imagination on your own, be sure to gather your own posse of safety as needed before engaging in dialogue with dream characters, objects, and landscapes. I have provided an exercise that explains how to do this in the coming pages.

If you do engage in active imagination on your own, it will help a great deal if you write or voice record the dialogue you create to keep you on track. This will help you find and retain the alternate voices of the dream that were not there when you first dreamed it. It is fine to go back and edit your reflections later on if you feel there are better solutions.

To illustrate dyad active imagination, here is dreamwork that my client Alisa and I did together. Alisa dreamed the following.

> *I am in a house with glass ceilings surrounded by big trees in a storm. The storm caused the trees to fall one by one and destroyed the house. I am scared because my son Peter is somewhere in the house. I finally find him, and he is all right. Once I find him, I am surprisingly not that scared or upset that the house is all broken down.*

One useful method to start dreamwork is to create a working title for the dream. Then, after the dreamwork is completed, you can revisit the title and see if it has changed. Usually it has, and the new title reflects the work and the healing or growth from the exploration. Alisa's initial title was "The Glass Ceiling." She had an immediate association with the phrase "glass ceiling," which is connected to women being held back from advancing in their fields of employment or politics by an invisible glass ceiling of gender inequity that stops their progression. This helped Alisa contextualize that the dream was connected to her work, specifically her challenges around how to be "bigger," to use her own voice more confidently and strongly.

Once Alisa titled the dream, we moved into active imagination work. I asked her if there was anything she needed to feel safe and protected at this point, and she said no, the storm had already passed. I invited her to connect with the dream and the central image of the house that was destroyed by a storm and to just see what came next. What did she want to do from there?

Alisa's first association to this house with the glass ceiling was that the old ways of being in the world were breaking down, no longer viable in this stormy season of upheaval all over the world politically, spiritually, and—specifically in relation to the storm—environmentally. Working from inside the dream, Alisa accepted that it is time for something new in her own life, which accounted for her relative lack of upset in the dream after she found her son. Then, Alisa said it was time for a new house to be built. When I asked her what she envisioned for her new house, she replied that the old house was too big, too hard-edged, and too cold and sterile with that glass ceiling anyhow, but that the ground floor was stable and made of quality wood. She decided that she wanted to take pieces from the ground floor and use them to build her new house.

When I asked her "What happens next?" (a good open-ended question to encourage the dreamer to engage in their own active imagination), Alisa replied that she would rebuild her house in the enchanted forest nearby and would journey to find just the right spot. My prompt was simply "Go ahead," as she was on a roll on her own and didn't need much more from me. She closed her eyes and narrated the following story as I jotted it down.

Alisa set out on her journey and came across a clearing in the woods with a waterfall, a stream, and mountains that felt just right. The forest animals and fairies that lived there came out of hiding and said to her, "We've been waiting for you. We will help you to build." It was a big project, and she recognized that she would need help with it. So, she and her

GAIA Method Applied to Ancestral Dreams and Nightmares

new helpers and her son went back to the site of the old house and began bringing beams of the wooden foundation to the new site. They laid the foundation of the new house with the quality wood floor that was left of the old one. This felt to her like a good place to stop. Alisa's new dream title was "Rebuilding."

Alisa and I didn't need to spend time establishing safety first because within the dream, the storm had already passed, she herself was safe, and she had found her son. However, it is still worth asking a dreamer if they'd like to establish safety. Alisa had been doing dreamwork and spiritual growth work for some time, so she was familiar with active imagination work.

It is not hard to see Alisa's dream as a soul journey, and she even used the word *journey* to describe her trek into the woods. Later, during the review phase, we made the bridge-to-life connection that Alisa had a good foundation in her own life: Her internal ground floor was solid and of value, so she didn't need to discard the whole thing. A house in a dream often represents the dreamer's body, the house of their soul—their home. Sometimes, this dream theme is structurally literal: the attic might represent your thoughts or mind; the bathroom, your own internal plumbing; the basement, your unconscious underground. Sometimes, this dream theme is more of a metaphor, as in Alisa's case. The ground floor of Alisa's dream house was a metaphor for the ground floor of her adult life, that is, her childhood and earlier life experiences. That was the base her life was formed on.

Alisa identified a stable-enough foundation to want to salvage and keep parts of it. There were parts of Alisa's childhood that were painful, that threatened at times to destroy her. One of her parents suffered from psychosis and was in and out of mental health hospitals for years. Those parts of the house were destroyed by the storms in her dream, and she was ready to move on and let them go. As she said right in the dream, she was not scared or upset that parts of the house were broken down. Sometimes, we need to break down to break through. The seed must shatter its shell to grow into the plant and flower.

From the moment Alisa engaged in the waking dreamwork of active imagination, her dream had fairy-tale and archetypical elements. She used her imagination to first visualize and describe what was in the dream and then what happened next, continuing the dream story actively in waking life. She found a clearing in the woods and was met by magical helpers, both animals and fairies. She got the help she needed, as she did not to have to do this work alone. She retrieved what was still solid and useful from her previous home.

The intergenerational piece was here as well, as Alisa was first frightened about her son, then relieved to find him, and finally built a new home together with him in a safer place where he could grow and thrive, this time with no glass ceilings. Alisa kept the foundational beams from her ancestors, retrieved them from the rubble left by the storm, and built anew for herself and her descendants with a posse of helpers that clearly transcended worlds and realities.

Active imagination encourages the conscious and unconscious minds to communicate with each other by directing attention and focus onto both the dreaming, unconscious self and the waking, thinking, curious self. I added the dreamer's ability to interact with the dream's characters, objects, and landscapes, as well as to their own somatic responses, to Jung's original formulation. You then have the ability to change the actions and outcomes that took place in your original dream by interacting with all the elements of it. You can go back and engage with various elements of the dream to create a safer, more satisfactory conclusion.

SEED Guidelines

SEED is a helpful acronym for doing active imagination work, either with dreams or in waking life. It is as follows.

See/Sense It: Visualize the images in your mind's eye; consider colors, shapes, sizes, background, and foreground; then add other senses such as sound, smell, taste, texture, or temperature

Elaborate on It: By using thick, rich descriptions, translate the image into language to access both sides of the brain

Embody It: Describe the image using a felt sense in the body; move and shape it in the body when applicable

Do Something with It: Move the image out into the world with some kind of action, whether it is actual, ritual, or symbolic; this could be small and simple or powerful and clear

The GAIA Method

The three stages of the GAIA method are:

1. **Preparation:** Pre-dreamwork preparation includes the gathering of multiple resources, with an emphasis on creating a felt sense of safety in the present moment, outside of the dream.
2. **The Bridge:** After the dreamer has connected with the resources from stage one, they peek into the dream itself to find resources not previously noticed when the dream was first had.
3. **The Active Dreamwork:** Utilizing the resources that have been generated in stages one and two, the dreamer works directly with the dream material, both from outside and inside the dream.

If you are working with guided imagery or stories from your ancestors that you are exploring on your own as opposed to dream material, many aspects of the GAIA method are effective as well.

Stage One: Gathering Resources and Allies

Prior to moving into active dreamwork with a frightening nightmare or engaging with an ancestor who frightens you or makes demands, you need to feel safe enough to interact so that you do not become triggered. This is the first step in all good trauma treatment approaches. Safety first. This stage is about slow and careful work to prevent abreaction or an anxiety response by building in resources to be able to tolerate the nightmares. As you do this work, use the same gentleness and compassion with yourself as you would with a cherished other. Practice slow titration.

The concept of titration is used in trauma treatment, though it was borrowed from the field of pharmaceuticals. A medicine dropper is used to titrate the correct dosage of a medicine, drop by drop. Similarly, by practicing titration, you inch into the experience and check your responses before adding more to the mix.

Here is an example of what this may look like. Let's say you are acting as a guide. When the dreamer tells you that they had a dream, ask them if they'd like to talk about it instead of assuming that they do. They may be ready, or they might just want to share that they were upset or unnerved by a dream that they do not want to work on right now. Respect whatever their pacing is, and only go as fast as the slowest part of them can safely tolerate. If the dreamer wants to talk about the dream, first share with them this protocol of establishing safety and protection so they will not be overwhelmed. Provide a brief overview of the window of tolerance, and check in as you proceed so everyone stays inside their window. Remember, it is okay to go to the edges of your window/comfort zone, but you don't want to overshoot into panic or shutdown.

If you are doing this work on your own, ask yourself if you are safe and ready before proceeding. Listen for the felt sense of "yes," for the green light. Once you get the green light, remind yourself that all dreams come bearing gifts, even the frightening or disturbing ones, and that if this dream involves your ancestors, the gifts yet to be discovered may be shared to heal past and future generations. Pre-supposing that there will be benefits from this exploration helps orient you toward healing. This then becomes the *kavanah*, or the intention of the work. When you point yourself in the direction you want to go, you are much more likely to end up in that place. So, when you orient yourself toward health and healing, you will then find it easier to achieve.

Next, ask yourself (or the dreamer) what the current title of the dream is. The title should be intuitive; don't overthink it. If the title surprises you, so much the better. Oftentimes, the title itself carries the main theme of the dream. In this way, you are more likely to get the body-wisdom at the core of the dream. (Later, after the dreamwork is complete, you will ask if it has a new title. The new title usually reflects the healing that has occurred in a concrete way, a clear and often powerful affirmation of the healing work that has occurred. I call this part of the technique "Title and Re-Title.")

Once the dream has been titled, rate your (or the dreamer's) emotional state in the dream on a SUDS (Subjective Units of Distress) scale of zero to ten, with zero feeling calm or neutral and ten being the worst distress imaginable.

EXERCISE
Safe Place Imagery

Safe place imagery is a gold standard in many healing modalities, and a good next step.

1. Envision a place that is perfectly safe. It could be a place you have been to, seen, read about, or imagined. Some dreamers find peace alone in nature, others in the company of family or friends.

2. Create a thick, detailed description of this safe place. Pay attention to sights, sounds, smells, tastes, and sensations. The more details you can provide, the more real and available it will be.

3. Check to be sure that the place is completely safe. There should be nothing lurking in the bushes or at the edges of the scene that is unsafe. For those with a trauma history or ancestral trauma, this step is particularly important. If there is something not quite right, rework the scene or change to a different one altogether that passes the safety test completely.

4. Remind yourself (or the dreamer) that a safe place can be imaginary as well as literal, and work together to find such a place if need be. The collaborative nature of creating this safe place with a trusted other can be healing and co-regulating as well. Lastly, adding or simply using the sapphire-blue light of protection (see chapter 1) can be very useful here and adds continuity to the safe setting.

5. Once you have established your safe place, keep it in mind so you can return there during the subsequent work as needed.

I first did a version of this exercise in my early thirties, and I still use the image I came up with then! At the end of the path in the woods in my parents' backyard, I see and hear the sound of the babbling brook. I feel the warm rays of sunlight streaming through the trees and see them shimmering on the water. I inhale the woodsy smell and feel the warmth of the sun and the coolness of the shade. I hear occasional chirps of the birds. As I sit on the ground, I feel my back supported by the trunk of the tree I am leaning against.

Even writing this, I spontaneously sighed and felt a sense of peace come over me. A spontaneous movement such as a sigh, yawn, twitch, or shudder is a sign that your body is releasing something, maybe tension that you didn't even realize you were carrying. Powerful stuff.

★ ★ ★

EXERCISE
Gathering Your Posse

Once you have established a safe place, you are ready to gather your support system.

1. Ask yourself (or the dreamer) who and what you need to feel safe. Start with people. Who do you feel safe and secure with? Who would you want with you if the chips were down or the woods were dark? You can choose real people, fantasy figures, or characters from a book or movie. These could be real people in your current life or from childhood; they may be alive in this world or have already passed to the other side. You can also choose mythical or spiritual beings such as gods, angels, guides, and shamans. You may even want to call upon the ancestral Bright Ones who are ready and waiting to offer their help.

2. You are not limited to people or spiritual beings; you can invite animal companions as well. Perhaps you fondly remember a pet that was your main comfort and connection and/or have a current pet that provides the same ser-

vice. Again, your safety posse can include real animals or pets and/or stuffed or imaginary ones.

3. Next, tune in to your own deep wisdom to write down a list of these guides. Here is where working with another can be helpful, because if you get stuck and can't come up with a list that feels sufficient, they may make suggestions or ask questions to elicit ideas. Again, participatory co-creation can add a felt sense of safety to the process.

4. Double check to make sure that all these beings are completely safe for you. There should not be a hidden agenda or dangerous side to them lurking in the wings. If you find one, out they go! Only truly safe people in this posse.

5. Once your list is complete, ascertain where you want these allies to stand (beside you to the right or left, behind you, or in front of you) before entering the dreamwork.

Final Steps

To complete stage one of the GAIA method, ask yourself if you would like to bring any objects with you. Ancestral gifts or inherited objects may be welcome here, such as the coffee cup your grandmother always drank from, a braid of sweetgrass from your auntie, or the shirt your dad wore. Other objects that have made their way into the pantheon of protection have included a diver's suit that my client could easily zip into and a crystal given to another client by a healer he had worked with. Several people I've worked with chose religious or spiritual talismans such as a rosary or a chamsa. One client brought her cell phone, with all its features of calling, texting, GPS, and a flashlight for wayfinding in the dark dream. Another client, an enterprising twenty-something, made sure to bring her portable charger into the dreamscape along with her cell phone.

As with the safe place imagery, you want to get as rich of a description as possible of the people, animals, and objects in your support system. Getting all the details—color, shape, size, texture, sound, smell, feel, etc.—makes that support more real and therefore more available to you. For example, when one of my clients said she would bring her cat, not only

Chapter Seven

did she describe him to the last whisker, she also pulled out her phone and shared pictures of him.

Before moving on to stage two, you might want to ask yourself (or the dreamer) how old you were in the dream and get safety and protection for the youngest parts that are there. This is an important question in general for dreamwork; your dreamed self may not be the same age as you are currently. Your age inside the dream helps contextualize the dream's time frame. A younger version of you may have very different needs than the adult version of you describing the dream. Young parts might want a teddy bear or blankie. (If you introduce the GAIA method to children, these may be their first items on the list.) If your younger part has a comfort item that they carry around with them, be sure to invite it/them to join the dream posse.

To wrap up stage one, just keep on asking, "Anything else? Do you need anything else to feel safe and ready to address the dream?" until you get a clear "ready" response, either from yourself or the dreamer. This is a crucial step and is a hallmark of both dreamwork and trauma treatment. It is reasonable to feel a bit uncomfortable when journeying thorough pain and fear, but you should not feel unsafe again. This should be a different experience than the traumatic event; there are no brownie points for gratuitous suffering. Do not proceed to stage two until you get the green light.

Not all dreamers need every step listed here, but it is good to check. Some people are shy or reticent, others are defensively competent, and still others may need encouragement to ask for and create what they need.

Stage Two: The Bridge, the In-Between Transition Step

Before diving into the dream itself, take one more preliminary step. Here, on the bridge between the prep work (stage one) and the active dreamwork (stage two), you (or the dreamer) should stand on the threshold of the dream for a moment and peer inside.[68] Having gathered your posse of helpers and protectors, your objects, and your safe place, look inside the dream to see if there is anything else that can ground you, keep you safe,

---

68. I appreciate my colleague, Leslie Ellis, who had the seed idea for the bridge stage of the GAIA method.

or be a resource for you right inside of the dream. You may have missed something before, or maybe you saw it but didn't recognize its importance because you were focused on the active parts of the dream. Your wise unconscious may have provided you with options for healing and safety that are just waiting to be recognized by your conscious mind.

This prompt may be something like, "Now look inside the dream from outside of it and see if there is something you may not have noticed or neglected to mention before that is a help or resource. There may or may not be something, but look for it now." People tend to see what they are looking for, so this orients the brain's neural networks in the direction of healing.

This step is very empowering because it has the potential to allow you (or the dreamer) to connect with resources that were already there, already inside, just waiting to be noticed or discovered. When someone has been through trauma, their focus is on survival, and they don't always recognize how they got from threat or danger to safety and calm. The bridge allows you (or the dreamer) to reclaim pre-existing internal resources, even if you didn't immediately notice them. On second glance, one client found a gray-haired woman with long braids sitting quietly underneath a tree. Another client, whose dream involved flailing in the ocean and fears of drowning, heard a squeaking sound and turned to find a pod of dolphins swimming toward her. The dolphins then lifted her up and swam her to shore.

Stage Three: Working Directly with the Dream

Now that you have set the stage for safety and containment, it is time to begin working with the dream. This can be done from the outside the dream or inside of it. Neither is better than the other; they are simply different approaches. You (or the dreamer) may want to use both styles on the same dream, or you may choose the one that fits your dream and state of mind at this time.

Sometimes, dreamwork is done chronologically. Other times, people start at the strongest point, or the safest, or even the scariest if they have done a lot of prep work. There are many methods of dreamwork you can use.

Chapter Seven

Outside the Dream

If you (or the dreamer) choose to work from outside the dream, you will engage in a more cognitive style of analyzing it. Unpack the symbolic and metaphoric associations you (and others, if not doing this work alone) may have. Then, make connections to your life. What are you reminded of? What are the metaphors, archetypes, associations with fairy tales or myths, fun puns, plays on words, etc.? How do you make connections between the dream to your current life? Your younger self? The lives of your family members and ancestors?

A talent in dreamwork is the talent for association. Start with casting a wide net, and as you get clarity and resonance, draw the net in and keep the associations that have meaning for you.

EXERCISE
Sunray Association Circle

One way to unpack the symbolic and metaphoric association in a dream is to create a sunray association circle.

1. Pick the image you are working with. Write it on a piece of paper and draw a circle around it. Then, make rays like those extending from the sun. I recommend starting with six rays—you can always add more!

2. At the end of each ray, write an associative word or phrase.

3. When you have finished, go back and circle the words or phrases that resonate most strongly with the image in the dream. Here is where your paydirt will be!

Here is an example of a sunray association circle using the presence of a cat in a dream.

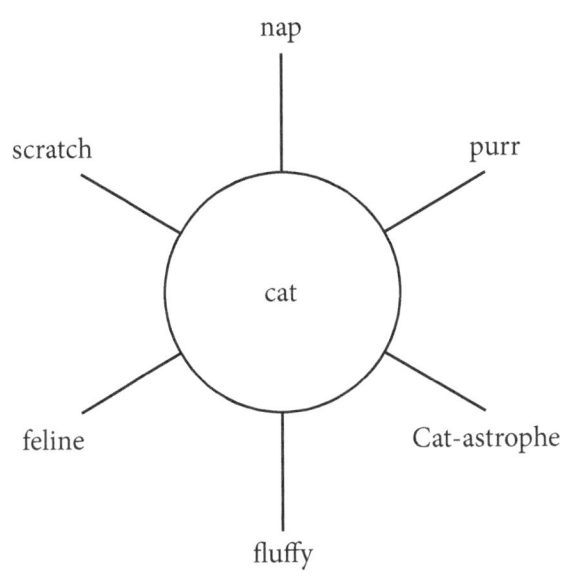

```
        nap
scratch       purr

       cat

feline       Cat-astrophe
       fluffy
```
Sunray Association Circle

Depending on which words you circle at the end of the rays, this exercise may indicate a lovely image, a scary image, and/or a time-marker that lets you know that the dream has something to do with your childhood. If I circled *purr, meow,* and *nap* in this example, that would be a very different dream cat than someone who circled *catastrophe, scratch,* and *allergic.*

* * *

How do you then make connections between the dream language and symbols and your waking life? And, once you have made connections, what do you need to do with this new information? Taking an action step following dreamwork is the key to transformation. The action doesn't have to be something large; it can be small and symbolic. Something like planting those flower bulbs, calling that relative you haven't spoken to in years, or making a donation to a cause changes your life in a much more concrete way than simply saying, "Oh yeah, I had this dream…" In this way, you put your dreaming knowledge to work to change your life.

Inside the Dream

Another way to work with a dream is from the inside. This is in the style of active imagination, where you re-enter the dream in your mind's eye and move inside of it as if you were still dreaming it. You interact in real-time with the characters and the landscape, asking questions and receiving replies that were not in the original dreamscape. You actively imagine what else might have happened or been said in the dream.

You also have the option of using the Gestalt method of dreamwork, where you can become every character—each animal, tree, rock, or hurricane in the dream—and speak as that voice. Who knows what you could discover if you acknowledged and became the flowering tree part of yourself, or the wild wind part of yourself, or the monster part of yourself?

Particularly when there is a danger or threat, allowing yourself to examine a dream from the point of view of that danger can open new worlds of understanding, self-healing, and ancestral healing. Because you are sufficiently safe and protected thanks to your preparation in stage one, you can now talk with the threat, have a dialogue, and see what is needed here. Have they been chasing you with a gift that you have been unknowingly running from, or do you need all your protections because the threat is full of rage and violence and needs to be healed, transformed, released, or banished?

I encourage you to read Mary Oliver's short poem about a box of darkness. It is titled "The Uses of Sorrow."[69] I was delighted by the first line of the poem, which tells readers that Oliver dreamed the poem while asleep—how appropriate! Remember, Pandora's box of darkness held all the world's pain and suffering, but at the end of the story, it also held hope.

Re-Dreaming the Dream

Once inside the dream, you can re-dream parts with your new resources. I call this *re-dreaming*, and I often tell the dreamer, "This isn't necessarily where the dream ended; it is just where you woke up. Now, you can continue dreaming the dream in a waking state. So, what happens next? And after that? And how would you like it to resolve?" This is also active imagi-

---

69. Oliver, *Upstream*.

nation. If you can imagine a new resolution, a new ending, and then repeat and review it, that new ending will become embedded in your psyche as a healing rewrite. The adage of "use a word three times and it's yours" applies to re-dreaming as well. Repeat the new evolution and ending three times, and you will have changed neural networks and made progress on transforming the dream and what generated it.

Leila's Dream

In this example, I used the GAIA method to help a client work with a nightmare.

Leila was a seventy-five-year-old Armenian woman who had been plagued by nightmares and somatic sleep disturbances for several decades. Her adult daughter brought her in to see me because Leila could not shake her repetitive nightmares. Extensive medical work-ups found no organic cause, and despite traditional and herbal medicine trials for sleep aid, Leila continued to suffer. She described waking in the night with heart palpitations, sweating and feeling terrified. Frequently, Leila couldn't get back to sleep, so she was fatigued during the day. She reported that these nightmares, which had persisted for years, were always the same or very similar.

History

Contextualizing Leila's background helps us understand how her dreams related to her life. Leila's parents survived the Armenian genocide in the early 1900s. As a young woman, Leila herself survived a terrible earthquake in Armenia and witnessed the building across the street from her completely collapse, killing all inside. Leila reported that she had wanted to follow her parents into a career in the performing arts but instead, she ended up marrying young and had two children. Shortly thereafter, Leila and her family left Armenia and moved first to Russia, then to America, where she raised her children. With this history and context, it is apparent that Leila had several displacements, traumatic upheavals, and losses in her life.

There were two common themes in Leila's nightmares. One theme was that she was being followed and chased by some men on a particular street in her hometown, and she was frightened that they would catch her. When I asked what they had been trying to do or tell her for so many years, Leila replied that they wanted to kill her. The other theme was that she had lost her way. In both sets of nightmares, it was dark, and Leila was worried that she had done something wrong.

Next Generation in the Room

I met with Leila and her daughter, who translated between Armenian and English, as Leila's English was not sufficient for complex, nuanced conversations. This added a whole layer of interest and challenge to our dreamwork, as not only did I have to pay attention to the dreamer herself, but to the translator as well.

Sometimes, I needed to clarify my question or comment to Leila's daughter first so she could reliably translate my meaning as well as my words while her mom worked on her dreams. The same process occurred in reverse, as Leila's daughter conveyed to me her mother's layers of meaning as she understood them. We were doing intergenerational healing work live in the room as well as within the dream. Not surprisingly, Leila's daughter had her own associations and somatic reactions to her mother's dreams and dreamwork.

Attending to the Body

I found that paying extra special attention to Leila's facial expressions and body language helped me know if she had an aha moment or not, even before I got the translation. This is something that I do anyway as a somatic practitioner, but watching for the micro movements and breath changes helped when we were literally not speaking the same language. I did the same with her daughter, watching if anything her mom said registered with her in her body before she translated it into English.

We know that translation is almost by definition imperfect, so I wanted to get the nuances in both languages as best as I could. When doing dreamwork, we were already translating from the language of the unconscious to the language of the conscious and could lose something in that translation as well. Think for a moment about your own dreams. How often do you see something so clearly in the dream, yet have trouble describing it when you are awake? It is, in part, a problem of translation.

GAIA Method Applied to Ancestral Dreams and Nightmares

GAIA Stage One: Safe Place and Gathering Resources

Because of the level of upset connected with Leila's nightmares, I want to help her achieve a sense of safety in the moment before diving into the upset of the dream itself. Prior to doing direct work on her nightmares, I used a variety of energy psychology and cognitive interventions over a few sessions to help with her anxiety and sense of hopelessness.

When we did a safe place imagery, Leila recalled a special church from her childhood in Armenia that gave her a feeling of peace and comfort. She recalled what it was like approaching the church from the outside, where she would sit when she was inside, and what she saw around her. I invited her to practice going there in her mind's eye daily, particularly before going to sleep at night, and tuning in to where she felt that peace and comfort in her body.

I also asked Leila if she had any idea what her nightmares were connected to or were reflecting, but she did not. I explained how the GAIA method of dreamwork works, and it took a while of translating back and forth for her to understand that stage one of the method addressed the dream content, albeit slowly and carefully. She was anxious to get going already! But before turning around to face these shadow figures—to ask them who they were and why they were chasing her—she understood that she first must be safe and protected.

Not being able to see the shadow figures clearly within her dream was part of the problem. Leila finally identified that she needed light for protection since the street was so dark that she couldn't even see who was chasing her. She then identified that she wanted it to be daylight, specifically "dawn on the horizon with the bright light of the emerging sun creeping up into the sky." This was a good, clear specificity to make it real and alive for her.

With some prompting, Leila also realized that she needed a fiery circle of protection around her that could keep everything that was dangerous outside of it. Finally, she wanted wings to fly so that she could soar above the street and fly away if needed. With these images, objects, and new powers, she was ready to safely enter the dream to see what it was about.

Light and wings are the themes of Leila's preparation. We will shortly see how they reoccurred in the resolution of these nightmares.

GAIA Stage Two: The Bridge

I asked Leila if she would peek into the dream using the bridge, but there was nothing else she saw for protection, so we moved right into stage three.

GAIA Stage Three: Entering the Dreamscape

I invited Leila to gather her resources around her and enter the dream. Leila closed her eyes, and as she did, she shuddered. Before I even had a chance to intervene, she was angrily asking the dream men, "Why are you following me?"

Not wanting her to feel scared or unsafe as she habitually did in her dreams, I asked her if before talking with them, she could take a step back and look around to see if she could identity the street, if it was a place she had ever been before. She said "Oh, yes!" It was a street she recognized from when she was in her twenties. Before she was married, she took a bus from this street to work.

Finding the right pacing and rhythm of the dreamwork between dreamer and guide is crucial: not too fast, but not too slow either. This means that Leila and I dialogued back and forth to find the balance.

Leila told me that her father used to warn her and her siblings about this street, that it was the street that ghosts chased him down. She said her father used to say "Watch out for the ghost" every day before she went to work. She had no idea why. Leila said, "I don't know why this has stuck with me all these years, but it has."

I wanted to make sure that this new twist was not an error in translation, but her daughter said it was not an error, the right word was in fact *ghost*. Leila reconfirmed this in English as well. So, now we knew that the shadowy men chasing her were the ghosts her father had warned her about. Now that she could see them clearly, they were in fact "short little men," or dwarfs. This is another flavor of a common fairy-tale motif that can appear in our dreams, another layer connecting us to the greater world mythos.

With this new information, we had a road forward. First, these nightmare villains were not even hers, but something she inherited from the legacy of her father. He was no longer alive to ask who or what his ghosts were, but as a persecuted minority in his country, there could have been multiple associations for him. Second, what was true for Leila was that none of her family had lived in Armenia for over forty years, and whatever historical ghosts had been pursuing her father there were not a part of her own life in America, and certainly not now, if they ever were. As I shared this perspective with her, she agreed that these ghosts were not hers and not real.

I asked her the question I ask everyone who suffers from intergenerational trauma: *Is this yours to hold or carry?* Her answer was no. So, we created a plan to send the ghosts back over the veil, to the light of the beyond. They no longer belonged in this world. Leila was able to speak to the ghosts and tell them that she was freeing them so they could finish crossing over, finish their journey back, stop pursuing her, and be healed themselves. The ghosts then told her that they had gotten lost and had not been able to find their way home.

Here the second theme of the nightmares emerged: the being lost theme. It turns out that it was not Leila who was lost, but the ghosts from her father's life who were still haunting her. Because they had lost their way, she gave them wings (maybe sharing the ones she had envisioned for herself in stage one), oriented them to the light—in this instance, through the upper left corner of my office—and sent them over. On the count of three, Leila exhaled and breathed the ghosts over and out, telling them as she did so, "Goodbye. Go in peace and with blessings, and leave me alone now."

Following this final piece of dreamwork, I gently let Leila know that her active dreamwork brought healing not only to herself, but also to her father and whatever the ghosts of his past had been that haunted him in his life and his death. Leila had now protected her daughters from inheriting these specters as well. One of them shared this journey with her in real time and planned to share details with her sister.

I recommended that the final action step for Leila could be to go home and light a candle in her father's memory for the light of healing. She looked calmer and at peace, and when I asked if there was anything else she needed, she said, "No, everything is okay now."

We didn't have another meeting scheduled, but I followed up with her daughter via email. Leila's daughter told me that her mother was sleeping much more soundly and not waking up with palpitations or night sweats anymore. No more ghosts.

Healing Responses

Trauma survivors need to learn to be the center of their own personal narrative, not a character in a story from their past or their ancestor's past. Discerning what is yours, what is not yours, and what needs to be healed and let go of is a key part of this journey. That is what Leila did.

Somatic practitioner Peter Levine writes, "Trauma amplifies and evokes the expansion and contraction of the psyche, the body, and the soul. It is how we respond to a traumatic event that will determine whether the trauma will turn us to stone like Medusa or take us along a journey of vast and uncharted pathways as a spiritual teacher."[70] In the Greek myth of Medusa, after being slain by Perseus, Medusa's blood is taken in two vials. One vial had the power to kill, and the other contained the power to heal. The message here is that trauma resolution is a blessing of great power.

> **EXERCISE**
> ### Using the GAIA Method
> Take a moment to decide if you have a scary dream or nightmare to resolve. I recommend choosing one that involves family members or ancestors in some way, but you can practice this method with any dream, even if you are not sure of the familial or ancestral connections yet. If you work with the intention that your dreamwork will be multigenerationally healing or connecting, it will be. Alternatively, if you are comfortable and have some experience in this kind of work, offer to be a guide or touchstone safety person for someone else.
>
> Some dreams you can work on alone, and even though you are unlikely to get all the juice out, you can at least get started and then decide who you want to share the additional layers of meaning with. Other dreams, because of their level of upset or because they are classified in your mind as a nightmare, should

---

70. Levine and Frederick, *Waking the Tiger*.

not be attempted without a good support system. That support may be your dream circle, your partner, your therapist, your dream coach, or a close friend. Please don't be righteously uber-independent. You deserve help, and the way to counterbalance neglect and trauma from the past is to have caring others with you as you work, because they may be able to support you in ways you did not have when the trauma or dream happened.

If you want to do this exercise on your own, start with a nightmare that is relatively mild, no more than a five on the SUDS scale of distress. Bring in your posse of helpers and guides for accompaniment.

1. Once you have decided which dream you would like to explore, rate your dream from zero to ten on the SUDS scale of distress when you put your attention on the dream; zero is calm and relaxed, and ten is the worst distress you can imagine. If you give your SUDS a five or more, don't try this on your own. Gather at least one other person to support you in this journey.

Stage One: Pre-Dreamwork Safety Protocol

2. When you feel ready, ask yourself, *Who and what do I need to feel safe and protected enough to address this dream, or this part of the dream, or to go back inside the dream?* Look to people alive or dead, real or imaginary; animals of all kinds; or spiritual beings. Double check to be sure you are completely safe and these are the right supporters for you now. If not, bid them farewell and try again.

3. Consider the details of each resource. Get a rich, detailed description of each one to make them full-bodied in your imaginal space.

4. Keep asking, *Is there anything else I need to be perfectly safe?* I can't emphasize enough the importance of this preparatory work. Be cognizant of the difference between "unsafe" and "uncomfortable"; it is okay to feel somewhat

uncomfortable when doing challenging work, but it is not okay for you to feel unsafe.

5. Find out how old you are in the dream and how old you feel in the dream as you retell it—they may not be the same. Get the protection that the youngest part of you that is present needs. Look for time markers to give you a clue (the clothing you or others are wearing, what era it is, the other people in the dream, etc.).

Stage Two: The Bridge

6. Before diving inside the dream, you may want to peek into the dream and see if there is a resource there that you did not notice before. Often, if you look around, you'll find a previously undiscovered resource hiding in plain sight inside of your dreamscape. This step can be done from outside the dream looking in, or you can gather up the resources generated in stage one and enter the dream with them to look around before doing anything else.

Stage Three: Working with the Dream

7. Begin the process of dream reentry by determining where the best place to enter the dream is. Gather your safety people and objects. When you are ready, go ahead and enter the dream.

8. If you are ready to continue, what happens first? Next? What do you want to do/say? What do you need to stay safe? Does anyone in the dream (including you, dream ancestors, or other characters) need to apologize, make amends, give a blessing, or say "I love you"? Who needs what here? Can you make that happen using your dream reentry skill set? Anything else?

9. Is there anything else you need to say or do to feel complete? If working with a guide, they can offer ideas or suggestions if you are stuck, which you can accept or discard.

GAIA Method Applied to Ancestral Dreams and Nightmares

10. What happens when you add resources and action steps to the dream?

11. Is there any place in this dream that still feels unsafe or unfinished? Check carefully.

12. When you dream the dream forward, how does it end or resolve now? Rehearse and practice the new ending at least three times to embed it in your neural pathways.

13. How are you feeling now, compared to when you started the work? What bodily sensations do you have that might be connected to your feeling state?

14. Gather up the gifts you received from this dreamwork—the words, objects, writings, and learnings you now have. Make a list. Some learnings may be in writing, but others may need to come through as pictures or sketches.

15. As you prepare to leave the dreamscape, gather your learnings in a way that serves your highest purpose and is in the service of your growth and healing.

16. When you are back out of the dreamscape, ask yourself, *What did I discover? What has changed? How are my ancestors who showed up in the dream doing? Is there anything else that feels incomplete or not safe? What is my SUDS now? Has the title of my dream changed?* And finally, *How will I incorporate these learnings and action steps into my life today?*

EIGHT

YOUR ANCESTRAL TASKS: HONORING, HEALING, RETURNING, REMEMBERING

> Dark times are not rare, but that we have a right to expect some illumination...This illumination is less likely to come from ideas, but from human beings who kindle a light with the way they live their lives. When we remember those people who illuminated our lives, it can light us up again and again.
> —*Hannah Arendt*, The Human Condition

What are your ancestral tasks? Well, it depends.

What is yours to keep and to honor and to carry forward? What belongs to the past and needs to be healed and returned there? What is not yours to keep and needs to be not only released, but banished or transformed? How do you make meaning of your life and the lives of your ancestors, and how do you contextualize that meaning in the past, the present, and the future? How do you integrate your past and release it at the same time? How do you separate your past from your present life while still honoring it? Hard but crucial questions.

Some years ago, I had a client, a black woman named Josephine, who originally came to therapy for general relationship issues but soon moved into talking about the microaggressions and racism she was experiencing as a professor at a local university. She began to have a series of dreams about slaves shackled on an auction block, waiting to be sold. While she didn't recognize their faces, Josephine knew that they could have been her ancestors in the 1800s; her family had moved north from the deep south three generations prior. If the individuals in Josephine's dream were not her direct ancestors, then they were certainly part of her ancestral lineage.

Josephine realized that these dreams were triggered by her present-day experiences. As a black professor at a predominantly white university, she knew that her life, experiences, and opportunities were vastly different than her ancestors', yet she still experienced the looming shadows of ancestral slavery in her dreams. As we worked on her dreams, offering healing and blessings to these souls, she recognized that they needed to be remembered, and their stories needed to be told. Josephine believed that she owed it to herself and to her ancestors to find ways to move into her own sense of agency as a strong black woman and to challenge the repression she still experienced.

In the book *It Didn't Start with You*, Mark Wolynn recommends offering some healing sentences to the ancestors. Depending on your relationship with your departed, their needs, and your needs, you might open with these sentences, or you may weave them into conversation.

- "What happened to you won't be in vain."
- "I will honor you by living my life fully."
- "Now I understand what happened to you. That helps me heal too."
- "I will use what happened to you as a source of strength for me and my children."
- "I will make something good out of this tragedy."
- "I promise not to perpetuate the pain or suffering."[71]

Josephine embraced several of these powerful phrases, and they became part of her activism and her daily meditation. She remembered to use her breathwork and meditation skills to stay centered and calm when choosing to address the microaggressions she experienced. As an action step, she volunteered to chair the school's BIPOC student group.

Jungian scholar Sandra Easter summarizes her own ancestor work into two core questions: "What is being asked of me now?" and "What needs

---

71. Wolynn, *It Didn't Start with You*, 147.

to be tended?"[72] Your ancestors carry your story, whether or not you know what it is, and you need each other to heal and repair.

Time and Timelessness with the Ancestors

In one of Moses's final speeches, he addresses his community of wanderers. But Moses doesn't speak only to those who are standing there with him. He does not say "all people," but "all those," which leaves the door open to all beings and other life forms. Moreover, he speaks of "those who are not here today," believed to imply future generations as well.[73] This sense of timelessness is referred to in many spiritual traditions. For example, there is the Lakota phrase *Aho Mitakuye Oyasin*, "all my relations," which has much the same meaning or implication: All life is sacred and timeless.

If you reach out to all your relations, who do you get? More than likely, you will access ancestors who are known to you and who are as of yet unknown. Lineage that you did not know of consciously will be illuminated when you reach out and remain open to these connections.

One somatic style teaches that connecting to your magical, ancestral ecosystem can help you transmute shame into power; liberate your ancestors from systemic oppression, ancestral woundings, and intergenerational trauma; and unlock your own true potential.[74] We know from trauma treatment (and therapy in general) that owning what happened reduces shame. When you can say to yourself, and/or on behalf of your ancestors, "Yes, this happened, and I am so sorry. How can I help now?" you are affecting a great transformation of power and healing.

Every night when you dream, you have an opportunity to cross the thresholds of consciousness and unconsciousness, to travel from one realm to the other. In Kabbalah, this is called *yerida*: the dropping down, the descent, the plunge. You drop down in order to go up. The continuum of consciousness that I shared in chapter 1 can be condensed into three realms: the conscious mind, the unconscious mind, and the superconscious mind

---

72. Easter, *Jung and the Ancestors*.
73. Deuteronomy 29:15 (New International Version).
74. See Rubinstein, *Writing at Time's Edge*.

Chapter Eight

that connects us with the Source. Taking the time to connect with Source can help you better connect with and heal your ancestors.

EXERCISE
Reaching Out Through All the Realms

Take a moment to attend to your intention here. Is it to recognize, to honor, to connect, to find beloveds from other times and places, or something else? Get clear, then settle down.

1. Sit with your feet on the floor and your back straight. Take a few deep breaths. Then, call in and surround yourself with the sapphire-blue light of spirit, healing, and transcendence. This container of light will help you cross the thresholds of time and space and then return safely to your own time/space. Listen with your inner ears and see with your inner eyes to open the door to more realms than you have access to in ordinary consciousness.

2. If it feels safe and right, reach out to your ancestors. Allow yourself to simply notice what happens at each level of your being as you tune in.

3. What happens in your physical body when you reach to your ancestors? (You may notice sensations, temperature or muscular changes, nausea, a smile, lightheadedness, a wave sense, etc.)

4. What happens to your thoughts and cognitions? (You may notice unusual ideas or thoughts that seem to come from elsewhere, thoughts or beliefs that seem to belong to your parents or grandparents more than to you, an aha moment, etc.)

5. What do you notice on an emotional level? (You may feel sad, angry, calm, beloved, etc., for no apparent reason.)

6. What is your soul or spirit saying to you? How is it responding? (You may feel a sense of awe, yearning, connection, envelopment, etc.)

7. What does your energy body know, see, or sense? (You may notice shivers, frissons, tingles, waves of electricity, a sense of resonance, etc.)

8. Recenter and reground your mind/body in the here and now. Open your eyes and look around your space. Register current time markers, such as a clock, watch, cell phone, or calendar. Register space markers in the room or place you are in, such as what you are wearing, what you are sitting on, or what you can hear.

When you are done, take a few moments to record what you experienced. You can use your dream journal for this; just make note of the exercise so that you remember where these experiences came from.

Waking Dream Healing Through Time

Here's a time twist: We know that waking life experiences can mimic a dream state of consciousness, so it makes sense that waking experiences of unusual or uncanny events may be reflecting a familial pattern from the past or future. Let's follow this thread of timelessness in dreams and dreamish, waking-life experiences.

In this next story, a member of my dream circle, Lois, connected a waking-dream state of consciousness to trauma in her family. Dreams may come through via multiple levels on the continuum of consciousness. Sometimes dream circle members work on waking-dream states of consciousness instead of dreams that came in the night, especially when someone has had a drought of night dreams, as was the case with Lois.

Lois told the dream circle that she recently took her dog, Jacko, for a walk in a nearby park that was swampy and full of brambles. Somehow, Jacko got away and disappeared in the park. Lois called and called his name, but he did not return. Jacko had been on a long leash for training purposes, and Lois worried he may have gotten twisted in the leash and stuck. After about three hours of searching and calling his name, her panic escalated, and Lois called a friend who advised her to contact the animal rescue league. Two rescue league workers showed up twenty minutes later, and one of them had a drone. Between their tracking skills and the drone, they finally found Jacko, who was shivering, whimpering, and stuck in a swampy area. Lois named her animal rescue team her "Angel Rescue Guys."

Lois learned that when trapped, many dogs do not respond to being called; perhaps this is a primitive or feral response to the need to hide for safety. I extrapolated that this is true for humans as well. The shivering and whimpering dog brought back memories of Lois's family stories. Several of Lois's ancestors perished in the Holocaust. Hiding did not protect them, and as camp numbers were tattooed on their arm, they lost their names as well as their lives.

In dream circle that day, we worked with this waking-life event of losing her dog as we would work with a dream. Lois and the group swiftly made a connection between Jacko the dog and her young grandson, who was on the autism spectrum and frequently could not respond to human contact or vocal cues. At the beginning of each dream circle we have a check in, and Lois had been sharing her pain about her grandson for months, along with her feelings of helplessness and occasional panic. Had her grandson somehow become "twisted in the long leash" of old family epigenetics or patterns?

After Jacko's rescue, Lois took the follow-up action steps that are always encouraged in dreamwork. She wrote to thank the rescue team and made a donation to their organization. Lois's other takeaway from this waking dreamwork was to continue to help her daughter look for "Angel Rescue Guys" who could help her grandson. We ended our dream circle that day with a prayer for an angel to come help her grandson.

Two weeks after Jacko's rescue, Lois came back to dream circle and reported the best visit with her grandson she had had in over eight months. Lois's daughter had scheduled an appointment that resulted in an adjustment to his medication, and that change enabled Lois's grandson to interact with people in a way he had not been able to for a long time. With Lois's insights and actions, and with the support of her posse of dreamers, Lois made a dream come true.

Finding meaning and taking action after trauma, tragedy, or grief is central to recovery. Being able to do this while things are still ongoing in some way can give you a sense of self-efficacy and empowerment.

Responding to the Six Calls

As I shared in chapter 1, each of the six ancestral calls offers something or asks for something:

1. "I am still here, and you are not alone."
2. "Take these gifts, blessings, or apologies."
3. "Let me help, heal, or warn you."
4. "Please, please help and heal me; I am still suffering."
5. "Watch out: This old grudge has not yet been resolved."
6. "Carry on my name and gifts to your children and your children's children. Remember."

Calls one and six are two sides of the same coin: *We were, we are, and we continue; death is not the end.* Calls two and three also form a matched set. Sometimes the ancestors want to give us a blessing or gift. Sometimes they feel bad about what transpired in their embodied life and are asking for forgiveness. Sometimes we need their help, and they are offering it whether or not we asked. The ancestors see more than we can see from a singular perspective.

In call four, the ancestors are asking for healing. When they suffered a great deal in life, they need to resolve whatever hurts were not resolved when they died so they can fully go into the light. If ancestors died harboring hurt, trauma, or pain, the help we can provide will be a win/win on both sides of the veil.

Call five is about the healing of old grudges. This call may need a whole different set of interventions if these ancestors show up with demands. Here, the work may include ending the grudge and cutting off contact with those holding the grudge.

Let's look now at how you can respond to each call in a way that honors and serves the ancestors and your own highest purpose.

Chapter Eight

Message One: "I Am Still Here, and You Are Not Alone."

One of the most difficult parts of grief is the sense of loss associated with a connection no longer being available to us. The smell of a loved one may be missing, their belongings are no longer scattered around the house, and gone are the connective points such as talking, texting, taking a walk, or having a meal together. Being able to find new points of connection after death enlivens us as it enlivens the spirits of the departed.

Being and feeling accompanied in life are some of the best parts of having family and friends. To continue to have this accompaniment even after death is a gift we can receive *and* can look for and invite. The felt sense of a loved one's presence is still available to you if they can cross the veil. Some ancestors only show up if you issue them an invitation; others are already there, just waiting to be seen and recognized via signs and symbols or dream visits.

Marina, a member of my dream circle, lost her father a few years ago. She asked the universe for a sign that he was still around. After sorrowfully reporting for several weeks that she had not had any dream visits, she was thrilled to have received a sign—literally. While walking around, she saw a street sign with the name George Street on it. George was her father's name. Here was Marina's sign. Sometimes ancestors have a sense of humor. She could all but hear him saying to her, "Well, you *did* ask for a sign…"

Allow yourself the suspension of disbelief if you struggle with the idea of having an ongoing relationship with your departed loved ones. Gently set disbelief aside, and remain open to the possibility of connecting, even if you are not sure this is possible. People see what they look for and notice what they are seeking. So, let yourself see the signs too, even if they are not as literal as a street sign. Did your beloved show up in a dream? Did you see their name or a similar face out and about? Were you visited by a bird or another winged creature? Angels and birds both have wings; perhaps that is why birds are frequently messengers between worlds. Specifically, the owl is revered not only for wisdom, but also as the harbinger of messages from the dead.

If you are not receiving signs or symbols from a departed loved one, don't forget to issue an invite! Your polite ancestors may just be waiting for one. Say whatever is in your heart. An invitation may simply be "I would love a visit. Please let me know you are here."

After receiving a sign or symbol, be sure to acknowledge it by saying something like "Hi, it was so nice to see you" or "Thank you for visiting."

Message Two: "Take These Gifts, Blessings, or Apologies."

Sometimes ancestors want to offer us something that they did not or could not offer while they were alive. The offering may take the form of an object or a blessing, and the blessing itself may contain words, touch, or an energy transmission. An apology is usually something they wished they could have said before passing; this can go both ways.

After talking about ancestral dreaming with her dream circle, Joy had the following dream.

> There is a line of flying hearts swirling around me and my husband. They are a type of flying transportation. They fly over to us and attach to us. The hearts turn into millions of little pieces crawling all over my body and face, which feels creepy and uncomfortable.
>
> In the next scene, I'm observing a dance class to see if I want to take the class. I watch for a while, then I try to join in with some flying flips. Everyone is impressed. I try to fly home, but I'm not used to it and can't get enough height. I finally get the hang of it, and I'm flying down a darkened hallway toward home. All of a sudden it feels comfortable and familiar, as if this is what I'm meant to do.
>
> When I get home, my mom tells me it's my legacy from my grandmother who used to fly like that, and she would be proud of me for carrying on the tradition.

Joy believed the dream was about accepting gifts from her ancestors, even if it made her feel uncomfortable at first. She shared that the flying hearts told her these gifts were given in love. This dream also had a deeper meaning for Joy. After her mother died, her father wrote a parable about their relationship and children. He cast himself as a frog and Joy's mother as a bird. As much as the frog wanted to fly like the bird, he couldn't. Some of the children were frogs and some were birds. In her dad's story, Joy was one of the bird children, but she was too afraid to fly. Joy shared, "As I've gotten older, I've accepted my role in life. I can spread my wings and fly, and it feels like it's what I was meant to do all along!"

I was also curious about the flying hearts that became like little bugs that crawled all over Joy. Perhaps this metaphor is feeling "bugged" by things we need to accept when we are not willing or able to yet. They seemed to disappear in the next scene of the dream, and then Joy was willing to try to fly even though it was challenging. Finally, she got it. She accepted it. And if that wasn't clear enough, her mom told her right in the dream itself that flying was her legacy from her grandmother. When her mom told her that her grandmother would be proud of her, it removed any shame or reluctance, allowing Joy to carry on her traditions and work in the world.

I love this dreamer's progression from being uncomfortable accepting the gift of love and spreading her wings to realizing that it is her legacy and a gift bestowed. Your ancestors might bless you with things that surprise you, things you may not be up to, or things you feel you don't deserve. Sometimes you can resolve your ambivalence right in the dream, but other times you need to think on it and find a way to accept your blessing or task.

* * *

When my client Larisa's mother died after a short illness, she struggled with complicated grief because there had been years of conflict between the two of them. One night, Larisa had this dream.

> *My mom comes to me and says, "I'm so sorry for all the fights we had. I was so young when I became a mother, and I really didn't know how to do it and was always so worried about you. I want you to know that I always loved you, though."*

Here was the apology Larisa never got in life, and this dream visit made a big difference for her. Larisa was able to put down her anger and forge a new relationship with her mom through her dreamscape. She also began to practice automatic writing. After posing a starting prompt and setting a timer, Larisa allowed her unconscious to dictate what she wrote without editing. In the process, she found herself in dialogue with her mom, writing out both sides of the conversation. Larisa discovered things about herself and her mom that she was previously unaware of. This helped her contextualize her mom's temper in light of the fears and anxieties that she had inherited from her own mother.

It is common for us to repeat patterns we learned from our parents. I learned later in life that my mom had a lot of anxiety, but she took great pains not to show it to us kids. At times, she bent over backwards to do the opposite of her anxious instincts. For example, I was the first—and only—kid on my block who was allowed to cross a busy street to go to the convenience store, though I had to take my younger brother for company if I wanted to exercise this freedom. And my mom was afraid of the water, never having learned to swim since *her* mom and dad were fearful too. She made sure that my brothers and I all took swimming lessons from a young age. I do have my own anxiety legacy as well, but my mom did a good job recognizing that she had choices in her own parenting. Thanks, Mom!

Message Three: "Let Me Help, Heal, or Warn You."

In this call and so many others, the ancestors say, "Let me help you," and sometimes they add, "Then you can help others." Help and healing are two-way streets. Ancestors who were able to complete the healing they needed are now available to help you resolve issues or wounds in your own life. You may ask your departed loved ones for their opinions on a life choice, whether you should get a new job or a new partner, or something else that is deep in your soul. Whether in a waking state or a sleeping dream, you can request the assistance you need and open yourself to what they have to say. This is part of the premise of dream incubation as well.

The Trauma of Being Unseen

Neglect is trauma. Neglect can include the absence of the concrete needs of daily life, such as food and shelter, and the absence or lack of sufficient love, care, or good parenting. Not being seen or cared for when young can create a sense of emptiness or not-enoughness that can persist throughout life if not healed. Having a solid attachment and connection to a loving caregiver in early life is critical to developing a strong sense of self and solid self-esteem.

Luckily, we are all hardwired for healing, so this is possible even later in life. The importance of being witnessed is key. If you were not witnessed sufficiently by others as a child, developing your own inner witness can help you internalize self-knowledge and the state of being seen. Healing trauma is about restoring connection to yourself and to others. Living in equanimity within your own embodied self and living with community support your healing and the healing of your ancestors and descendants.

Many of my clients over the years have come to therapy to resolve issues of life transitions or choices, anxiety, and depression, but they frequently need to experience the sense of re-parenting that deep, long-term therapy can provide at its best. The ongoing gaze of love between a mother and child is called the nursing dyad. The infant is seen, loved, and fed while being held both literally and figuratively. I am blessed to have a black-and-white picture of myself as an infant with my mom leaning over me, beaming, as I reach for her chin. I can see the love there. This dynamic was often missing in the lives of those who feel they are not enough, or too much, or not worthy.

As I noted before, we parent the way we were parented unless we have gained the awareness to make healthier choices about what approaches to keep and what to discard. The intergenerational trauma of neglect and/or the lack of those crucial early bonding experiences can be transmitted from generation to generation until awareness or exposure heal this pattern. For example, several of my long-term clients wrote beautiful letters to me when we terminated our work, each saying in their own way, "Thank you for being the mother I never had." I was profoundly moved.

Rob's Story

My client Rob chronically felt that he was too much, taking up too much time and space. That was the message he got from his mother all throughout his childhood: "Quiet down. Don't bother me. Stop asking questions. Don't make waves." As an adult, Rob tended to overexplain (different from "mansplaining," as this was Rob's effort to be seen, heard, and understood rather than to control or instruct).

Rob shared that this lack of confidence in himself stemmed from both sides of his family. His scientist father was meek and quiet, and he gave up easily when there was a disagreement with his wife. Rob's mother was a professional, and she actually told her children that she didn't really want to be a mother, but that was the price of getting married to continue with her career. (Ouch!) In high school, Rob went through a period where he fell apart, then reconstituted himself with a drive to earn his parents' love by excelling in college. He never felt filled up emotionally, and trusting himself and others was always an issue. *Am I good enough? Lovable enough? Do I have enough? Am I enough?* were questions that haunted him.

To understand where this pattern came from in Rob's family, we began retracing his maternal line after acknowledging that this was where the painful pattern had its deepest roots. To start with a potential resource for grounding and anchoring, as in the GAIA method, I first asked Rob if there was anyone he knew or had heard stories about who was a loving mother figure on that side of the family. Rob replied that he had heard stories that his maternal grandmother Alice was a loving mother.

Here's what happened, though: Grandma Alice died when her daughter Barbara, Rob's mother, was only five years old. Apparently, the family blamed Barb for her mother's death, saying that she had "weakened her mother" during childbirth. So, Barb was left motherless at age five, then neglected/un-parented by a series of "wicked stepmothers" as her father remarried a few times. Barb was raised to carry a profound early loss and undeserved blame for the death of her mother. "Just buck up" was the message Barb received. She "bucked up" by focusing on academic success, not relationships.

We can see that Rob's family legacy of neglect and unresolved grief extended for three generations. Explanation is not an excuse, but it does help with understanding. To enhance Rob's healing beyond simply understanding, and to get closer to his soul-worth, I invited him to tune in to Grandma Alice in a guided meditation. After Rob closed his eyes, I said, "Allow yourself to see Grandma Alice. Look into her eyes and see her beaming her love to you. She is here for you now in the fullness of time and can hold you and love you as she did with her daughter. Allow yourself to be filled up with her love. See her seeing and loving you. Know that you are enough, and you are good enough. You are not too much just the way you are. Let this love ripple from Alice through time and space to your mom Barb so she too can receive her birthright of motherly love. Know that as you do so, and as you are filled up with this love and acceptance, you are doing the healing work for your whole family, including your younger self and your own children. You are now stopping this old pattern, so as you parent your children from the fullness of yourself, seeing their wholeness as well, it will resonate down through the generations. May it be so."

Never underestimate the power of good guided imagery in combination with a caring relationship! Rob had his hands over his heart and we both had tears in our eyes as we finished. Understanding the source of the hurt and pain allowed for forgiveness and compassion for all involved, and this work gave Rob new insight into parenting his preteen daughter.

When you retell your family saga as a sacred story, it becomes part of your healing rather than your suffering. In this way, you can learn the life lessons that your ancestors were not able to or did not have access to, and you can open doors that were closed because of so much pain. Psychotherapist Gabor Maté teaches that the wisdom from trauma comes when we realize that our traumatic responses and imprints are not us, and that we can follow all traumatic responses back to the source to work through them, let them dissipate, and reconnect to the consciousness we were born with.[75]

EXERCISE
Find Your Wise and Well Elder

Allow yourself to take the journey that Rob did.

1. Look at your genogram to find an ancestor who you identify as a loving, guiding presence. This may be a parent or primary caregiver, an aunt or uncle, a grandparent, a cousin, a sibling, etc. If there is no one you can identify, widen your field to include loving spiritual beings with whom you feel a kinship.

---

75. Maté and Maté, *The Myth of Normal*.

2. Once you have identified this person or being, reach out to invite them to partner with you and help you feel seen and known.

3. Ask someone to read this meditation out loud to you as you close your eyes, or read the meditation softly to yourself:

   Allow yourself to see your ancestor. Call them by name. Look into their eyes and see them beaming their love to you. Feel their beaming love throughout your body and soul. They are here for you now in the fullness of time and can hold you and love you with their best self.

   Allow yourself to be filled up with their love and know that you are enough, that you are good enough, just the way you are.

   Let this love ripple from your ancestor through time and space to the previous generation, your parents, so they too can receive their birthright of unconditional love. Let this love ripple to the next generation and your descendants. Know that as you do so, you are being filled up with this love and acceptance. You are doing the healing work for your whole family, including your younger self and your own children. You are now stopping this old pattern. As you parent your descendants from the fullness of yourself, seeing their wholeness as well, it will resonate down through the generations. Thank your ancestor for partnering with you and extending their love to you. May it be so.

4. When you have completed the meditation, write about it in your journal to preserve these messages.

Message Four: "Please, Please Help and Heal Me; I Am Still Suffering."

When ancestors die without the opportunity or the resources to resolve their pain or trauma, sometimes they get stuck in the in-between, not here on Earth anymore, but not fully at peace in the afterlife. They may be asking or begging for assistance, either in a shout or a whisper. When you help your ancestors, you help yourself and resolve the story they were stuck in, and you create a new story of wholeness and healing.

Energy of the Afterlife

Even if you don't have a belief system that includes an afterlife, we know that energy is neither created nor destroyed. On the most basic level, energy and mass (matter) are interchangeable; they are different forms of the same thing.[76] And since we have energy bodies as well as physical bodies, I can't help but wonder what happens to that energy when we die. My personal belief is a combination of science and spirituality: The energy that enlivened us when alive is still in the universe when the body dies. That energy then joins with the universal energy of Oneness while retaining the imprint of the being we embodied so we can be recognized by loved ones who are still alive.

An intergenerational spiritual perspective tells us that the energy of the ancestors is somewhere. And if they did not die in peace, their energy or spirit may still be looking for help resolving the tangles of pain so they may pass fully. They may need a variety of interventions. This next story combines a request for help with a request to remember.

Joy's Story

Joy, an author and illustrator of children's books, knew that her great-grandmother Rachel died in the Holocaust, but she did not know the details. Several years ago, Joy and her husband were on a river cruise down the Danube. Their first stop was Regensburg, Germany, where Joy did some research on the *Stolpersteine*, "stumbling stones," which memorialize Holocaust victims throughout Europe. After finding several stumbling stones in Regensburg, Joy and her husband returned to the ship.

Joy was jet-lagged, so she attempted to nap on the sundeck. In the high heat, she heard a voice in her head saying, *The death of Rachel.* Joy asked, "Rachel who?" and heard, *Ruchla—Ruchel Adler.* She recognized the name

---

76. "Introduction."

because Adler was the maiden name of her great-grandmother who died in the Holocaust along with her husband and two daughters.

Since Joy never knew the family's exact fate, she asked the voice if Rachel died in the death camps. The voice said yes. The voice was female, and Joy was beginning to suspect she may be talking to Rachel herself. She asked which death camp Rachel had died in and heard *Treblinka*.

Joy said she was sorry that Rachel had to endure that and then asked the voice what it wanted. The voice said, *Don't forget me*, and Joy said she wouldn't. Then, Joy asked if Rachel knew that she had submitted her name and the names of her family members to the Hall of Names Memorial at Yad Vashem, the world Holocaust remembrance center. The voice said yes, she appreciated that. Joy told Rachel that she wouldn't forget her and thanked her for the contact.

After Joy returned from her trip, she discussed the waking dream with her dream circle. One member said that Rachel sounded like she could be a character in one of Joy's books. Joy thought about that comment and decided to dedicate one of her upcoming books to her great-grandparents so that their names would be remembered by current and future generations of children.

Joy has a Hanukkah book coming out soon that will be dedicated to her great-grandparents. She even included a photo of them on the living room wall in one of the book's scenes. She hopes Rachel will be happy with the decision to include her great-grandparents in her book.

Sometimes the help an ancestor is asking for is to be remembered for their life, not only their death.

Message Five: "Watch Out: This Old Grudge Has Not Yet Been Resolved."

You may consciously or unconsciously carry old grudges from generations back, and your relatives can show up in waking life patterns and in your dreams with various demands or upsetting themes that you can't seem to shake. What better way to tap into your buried unconscious than through your dream life? You can use a variety of unpacking methods to sort out the dreams and free yourself of an old and unwanted inheritance.

Chapter Eight

Here is where the rubber meets the road, so to speak. You will need extra protection to do this kind of work, since these ancestors are not at peace and will disturb you and your peace to perpetuate their feuds. These are the ancestors who are still raging, who can't let go of old hurts and feelings of being slighted, ignored, or passed over. They may show up in your dreams as themselves or disguised as a wolf, werewolf, or monster of some sort. They may be chasing you or pop up in front of you on a dream road.

If you have had the courage to ask this kind of ancestor who they are or what they want, they may have told you that they still want revenge or want you to maintain a cut-off in your family as part of your legacy burden. You have the power of choice here. Are their grudges still relevant for your life today, or do they simply weigh you down?

Then, your work is to do your research and try to figure out what your ancestor is still angry about, what wrong they want righted, and where it began. Remind yourself that you are not your mother, brother, etc. No matter how this ancestor's legacy has touched your life thus far, you have the choice and the power to differentiate yourself from them.

Once you become aware of the grudge and recognize the hurt that fuels the anger, you can offer healing and forgiveness and tell a new story. Awareness of the source of the pattern will help you contextualize and let go once you realize that this grudge is not a part of your own life.

Here's a fictional story I heard at a workshop about an old grudge with an ironic twist.

> *A few years ago, the Miller brothers from South Carolina made a long, purposeful road trip all the way to Alaska to find the Smith family, a family they had feuded with since the Civil War.*
>
> *"The Millers always fought the Smiths," said one of the Miller brothers when they found the Smiths, "Ever since your great-great-granddaddy shot mine in the neck."*
>
> *After some discussion about when and how their own fight or duel should take place, Mr. Smith reflectively said, "Well, you know, if we fight this match now and one side clearly wins and the other clearly*

loses, we lose our whole reason for living. This grudge has been the raison d'être for all of us, so then what? If it is settled, what do we live for?"

"Hmmph, good point," was the response.

And with that, the men decide not to fight and to live for another day. Grudge match tabled, they reached a truce and moved forward.

While this might not be the only way to settle a grudge, it seemed to work here. Letting go of ongoing violence or hurt is key. End the enmity in your generation as peacefully as possible. Find something else to live for, as the Millers and the Smiths did. Perpetuating a grudge doesn't serve you or your ancestors. Instead, this is another opportunity to do healing work, and this time it requires very clear boundaries.

EXERCISE
Protection When Working with Angry Ancestors

Before you begin to engage with these ancestors, take a moment to protect yourself. This might be a good time to use stage one of the GAIA method—safety first.

1. Surround yourself with the sapphire-blue light of divine protection. Make it strong and thick and able to protect you in all realms.

2. Add your own items of protection. You might want an invisibility cape, or you might envision adding angel wings to your energetic body. Feel the wings emerge from your shoulder blades. Know that you can then wrap yourself in your items of protection against all dark or angry energies. You have the right of choice and the power to reverse the curse.

3. After this, set boundaries with them as needed.

Boundary Balancing

After you have protected yourself against angry ancestors, engage in boundary balancing, an energy technique based on the mind/body work of Dr. Judith Swack. It consists of a series of cognitive statements that

Chapter Eight

allow you to have 100 percent healthy boundaries that Dr. Swack originally delineated at five levels of being: the physical, the cognitive, the emotional, the spiritual, and the energetic.[77] My dream circle and I later added a sixth level: the dreaming level. For the purposes of this book, I've added a seventh level of ancestral energies as well.

It is useful to imagine the image of a cell to understand the five functions of a boundary. Imagine a cell wall as the equivalent of a boundary. It serves five functions:

1. It keeps things out, including toxins and anything that threatens the cell.
2. It lets things in, like food, nutrients, and whatever the cell needs for growth.
3. It keeps things in. Everything that is an integral part of the cell itself stays inside the cell wall, like the nucleus, the mitochondria, the DNA strands, etc.
4. It lets things out, such as waste products, energy, and damaged or injured parts of the cell.
5. It communicates with other cells, sharing information and function.

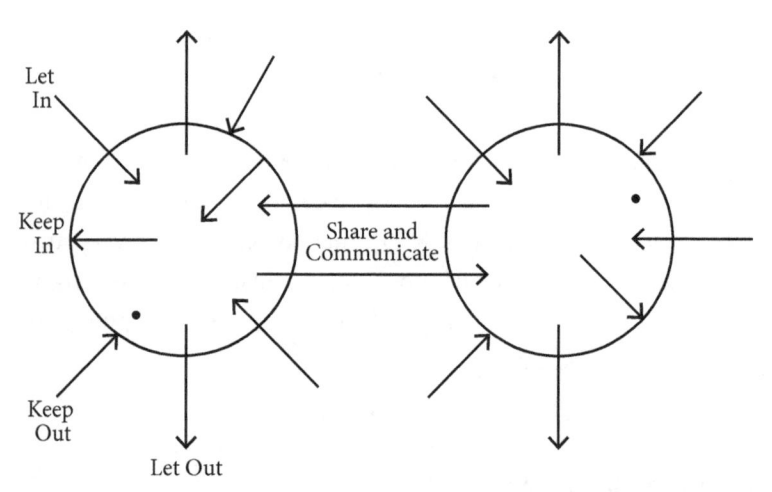

Five Functions of the Boundary Balance

---

77. Judith Swack, "Healing from the Body Level Up," workshop handout, April 14, 1997.

These are the same five functions that your energetic boundaries need to perform as well. We typically think of a boundary as keeping something out, but it is more complex than that. Both cell walls and human boundaries need to be communicative and permeable, opening and closing at the right time and with the right stimulus. And, as I mentioned, we need boundaries at all levels of being for optimal functioning:

1. **The Physical:** Who is physically with you; your own sensations; your physical integrity
2. **The Cognitive:** Your thoughts; your belief system
3. **The Emotional:** Your feelings
4. **The Spiritual:** Keeping your spiritual beliefs intact and not overly influenced by other peoples or entities from other realms
5. **The Energetic:** Not being influenced or hijacked by other people's energies or giving away too much of your own
6. **The Dreaming:** Letting in only the dreams and dream energy that serves you and keeping out the rest
7. **The Ancestral:** Keeping a clear line of demarcation between your life in a physical body and the departed, who are alive only in the spirit world

You can use muscle testing, also called *applied kinesiology*, to ascertain how many levels of intact boundaries you have at any given time. You can learn this technique from a practitioner of applied kinesiology, which can then be done with a colleague or friend, or on your own. Also, as an adaptation of this, simply ask yourself, *Do I have 100 percent healthy working boundaries between myself and X?* and listen intuitively for the answer to arise. The X might be nightmares, a particular person, uncontrolled upset or strong emotions from a nightmare, etc. If you get a "no" response, you can either move right on to the next exercise to reestablish your boundaries, or you can discern which of the levels might have been breached first.

EXERCISE
Boundary Balancing Technique

This exercise will involve tapping and/or feathering movements. You will intuitively decide which method(s) you need.

Tapping involves using one hand to gently tap your fingertips on your sternum in a spot that feels comfortable. If you prefer, you can tap the center of your chest, which corresponds with the central and governing meridians from acupuncture. Feathering involves taking the hand that was tapping on your sternum and gently moving it up your chest, up your throat, and out from under your chin, releasing your fingers at the end of each round.

1. If you believe your boundaries are not 100 percent intact, ask yourself how many minutes of tapping and/or feathering you need to reestablish healthy boundaries. Intuitively listen for the answer. Most people seem to need between one and five minutes, but you may need up to ten or fifteen.

2. If you'd like, bring in light with an angel. Invite an angel of your choice—who may or may not have a name—to bring you divine light. Notice what color(s) you need and then bring your hands up overhead, grabbing hold of the edge of the light shield and bring it down around your body.

3. Begin tapping your sternum and/or feathering your chest, throat, and chin. Repeat as needed until you have reached the allotted time.

4. While you are tapping and/or feathering, say out loud, "I have 100 percent healthy working boundaries between myself and X" (fear, a monster, your father, an ancestor, critical thoughts—whatever you need distance from).

5. When you have reached the allotted time, check to see if you now have 100 percent healthy working boundaries. If not, do a few more rounds.

Please know also that good boundary establishment is something you may need to do periodically or even regularly; it is not just "one and done." If you have chronic nightmares, you may need to do this nightly for a while. If you have a difficult family member, you might need to do it before you see them each time. Parents can use boundary balancing to avoid soaking up their children's angst and upset, and vice versa. With practice, you will tune in to when you need this balance more quickly. Tap your way to healthy boundaries!

★ ★ ★

EXERCISE
Sending Them Back

You might need a friend or therapist to support you in this exercise. Be sure you feel supported and ready to engage with an angry ancestor.

1. Once you have secured your boundaries, speak from the strong, determined, and protected part of yourself. Tell your ancestor that you are sending them back to the light, that their energy in this plane is done. They may protest, but that is not your concern. Think of the language you might use when parenting a toddler or teenager: "Yes, I understand that you want this, but no, you can't have it." What is needed here is a strong "no" on your part. Sometimes offering another choice works. In this case, the choice is simply, "You can go back to Source to heal on your own volition, or I can send you. Your choice, but either way, you are going and not staying in this plane any longer. This cycle of retribution is over."

2. You can give your ancestor a chance to share the roots of their enmity if you want, but it is not required. Be compassionate, but not at the expense of firm limits and boundaries.

3. When you are ready, send them back to Source. Call on the help of angels or spirit guides, if desired. Then, breathe in for a count of three. Strongly exhale with an audible "Whooooosh."

4. Then, because nature abhors a vacuum, fill the gap that is left by your ancestor's absence in your psyche with love and light. Don't neglect this step.

5. If you'd like, do some energy clearing using cleansing herbs such as rosemary or sweetgrass.

Message Six: "Carry On My Name and Gifts to Your Children and Your Children's Children. Remember."

Was the language of your ancestors passed down proudly, or was it hidden as a "secret language"? Did it bear the shine of pride or the scars of trauma? Was it used to hide a conversation from children? (My mother told us she knew she was being talked about when her parents spoke Yiddish.) Maybe now is the time to honor that language. Dust it off if it was buried. Learn a few words in your ancestors' mother tongue. Speaking their language is another way to honor and heal.

Tell your children, grandchildren, and great-grandchildren about their ancestors. Identify the artifacts and mementos you got from them. Start a fund in their name. Name your own children after them, directly or indirectly. Tattoo their names on your body to memorialize them. Speak their names when you offer a prayer. Make them an altar somewhere convenient for you to visit. Commemorate.

You will source your own story in the lives of your ancestors, remembering their names, then seeding them to your children and others. In doing so, you will make the story of your own life richer as you carry on the legacy of their memory.

What is the name you were given by your ancestors? In addition to your given name, is there a name are you carrying from their legacy? Is it Hope or Despair? Love or Hate? Fear or Courage? Rage or Compassion? Victim or Survivor? These, too, are inherited names you may be carrying in your body, mind, or spirit. You have the choice to keep or to discard these names.

Awareness brings choice. Grieve your beloveds and choose the healing road.

NINE

CONVERSATIONS, COMPASSION, AND CREATIVITY FOR ANCESTRAL HEALING

> In all things there is a hidden wholeness.
> —*Parker J. Palmer,* The Hidden Wholeness

You are rooted in the generations that came before you. The web of your ancestors weaves its silken strands through your life, as deep as your DNA. If you listen carefully to the various calls, you will be given additional opportunities to have the conversations you wish you could have had. You can be granted more time and connection with your loved ones. You can do your intergenerational healing work with compassion and a dose of humor to lighten the load. Trauma in your ancestors' lives may have obscured their grace and wholeness, but they are still there nonetheless. People may sometimes feel that they are broken, but they are not; the human essence is still whole.

A branch of Kabbalah that is based on the teachings of Isaac Luria, a sixteenth-century mystic, teaches that when the Divine formed the world, it created ten vessels to hold the light.[78] However, the vessels were too fragile, and they shattered and spilled the holy sparks of light everywhere. As the sparks scattered, they formed the cosmos and Earth. Humanity's task ever since has been to gather up and reunite these sparks, thus participating in healing ourselves and our world. This is a core teaching of

---

78. Adler, "Introduction to Kabbalah."

tikkun olam, repairing the world. By reuniting with your ancestors in a positive way, you are also reuniting your wholeness and the wholeness of the world. Each spark contains the essence of the wholeness from which it came.

Unprocessed pain can show up in your dreams, when the veil between worlds is thinner, or in unhealthy patterns in your waking life. For example, did your ancestors need to keep quiet and suppress parts of themselves for safety? Did hiding or silencing yourself become a pattern in your own life or in your family? You may have maintained survival strategies long past their usefulness. Is it now time for you to step into the wholeness and fullness of your voice and self. Do not hide away. When you reframe familial stories from victimhood to survivorship with compassion, conversation, and humor, you can heal forward and backward in time.

Conversations of Ancestral Healing

Isabel was raised in an upper-middle-class family with two professional parents: a doctor and a lawyer. From the outside, her life seemed enviable. However, Isabel's mother, Anne, frequently told the children that she resented having to care for them at the expense of her career. When Anne was drunk—which was quite regularly—she would sob and tell her children, "I am a terrible mother. I never should have had you. Leave me alone." Then, she would lie in bed with the shades drawn and the door shut for days or weeks at a time while the rest of the family tiptoed around.

By the time I met Isabel, she was a professional woman who didn't trust her own intelligence despite her graduate degree and successful career. She was divorced with two adult children. While Isabel's son was doing well, her daughter was struggling on many levels. Even though Anne had died two decades previously, part of Isabel's healing journey was her desire to move past the messages she received from her rejecting and mean-spirited mother, both for her own well-being and for her daughter's. She wanted to pass a different message to the next generation of women in her family.

In therapy, Isabel worked to rewrite her own narrative and to challenge the hurtful messages she had received from Anne. Isabel began to find and create new sources of mothering in waking life and in her dreamwork. Then, several of her dreams began to feature Anne as the main character, looking wraith-like, feeling intrusive, and menacingly reappearing. This reminded me of the concept of the "hungry ghost," an insatiable ancestor who has unfinished business in life. Hungry ghosts may come back to haunt family members if they are not properly venerated, appeased, and fed; they can also emerge if the deceased has been neglected or deserted by their ancestors.

Isabel decided to track down Anne's hungry ghost and find out why she could not pass over the veil into the light. But first, Isabel and I reviewed Anne's history. Anne had been orphaned at the age of two, and she and her sister were cared for by a resentful maternal aunt who never tired of telling them what a sacrifice she made by taking them in. "I never wanted two more children" was the message Anne heard over and over. (She had reported this story many times to Isabel.) In response to her aunt's resentful parenting, Anne made herself as small and as smart as possible and got out of her aunt's home by going to college at the age of sixteen. Fast forward a decade and Anne was a medical professional in the 1940s and '50s, a time when female doctors were rare. Having children was not part of Anne's life plan, but her husband wanted children as part of his showcase of success, and he made it clear that this was expected of Anne if they were to remain married. So, Anne found solace in the bottle whenever the burdens of her life were too much.

Isabel came to realize that her mother had been transmitting her own painful past. As we explored this history, Isabel saw many similarities to her own life and how she was parented. Like her mother, Isabel had one sister, and each of them had a daughter who could inherit this pattern if it was not transformed. In the therapy biz, we sometimes say, "Explanation, but not excuse." Anne was not able to find alternatives to this pattern, so she repeated it. However, the exploration of her mother's past led Isabel to greater empathy, understanding, and forgiveness. With this newfound understanding, Isabel was ready to confront the ghost of her deceased mother in waking dreamwork. We agreed to do it together in a session.

I asked Isabel to establish her own safety and protection first, and she grounded, centered, and called in the sapphire-blue container of light. Then, I invited her to visualize her mother from one of the many dreams she had had of her recently. I asked her, "Where is your mother?"

Isabel replied, "Both in front of me and inside my belly, solar plexus." (Notice this umbilical connection spot. This is the one place we should never retain connecting energy cords once the umbilical cord is cut; it keeps us from being fully our own person.)

"Are you ready to talk with her?" I asked.

Isabel said, "Yes." Then, to her mother, she said, "I love you. I understand you were hurt too, so I forgive you, but you can't stay inside me. You need to finish going over to the light."

"Ask your mother if there is anything she wants to say to respond."

Isabel channeled her mother's voice and said, "I'm sorry I didn't know how to be a better mother. I was so hurt. Please forgive me. I do love you." Then, Isabel replied, "Thank you. I forgive you and love you too, but now it is time for you to go so you can heal."

I said, "With the power of the sapphire light, go ahead and push her out of your body and into the light of the beyond, where her spirit can heal. Be sure to get all the attachments and cords that she is holding on with. Assure her that your forgiveness and love will follow her."

This process took a few tries. It seemed that Anne was afraid to pass over the veil, and her guilt was keeping her tied to this world and to Isabel. I suggested that Isabel reassure her mother that her true home was with Spirit, not on Earth, and that she would remember her and honor her memory. With this final message, Anne seemed ready to complete the process.

I said, "Now is the time to speak any last questions or words on either side, because once she is gone, you can't call her back. When you are ready, take three big breaths and exhale each time with a whoosh sound."

Isabel did this, spontaneously adding sweeping hand movements as well. Then, Isabel reported that she saw a shadow leave her body in the vicinity of her solar plexus and exit through the ceiling in the corner of the room. With the ghost of her mother released, Isabel felt that she could now offer her own daughter love and care without the shadow of childhood pain. Isabel could parent from a different place: one of forgiveness, understanding, and wholeness. She could help her daughter heal without this family legacy burden.

In Isabel's dialogue with the ghost of her mother, they were both able to say, "I'm sorry. Please forgive me. Thank you. I love you."

EXERCISE
Apologies and Appreciations

Take a moment to think about the people in your life, past and present. Think, too, about the land you live on or are connected to via your ancestral history. Are you aware of any nightmares connected to relatives? Are any stories of bad blood, grudges, unresolved arguments, or issues still binding you, taking up space in your mind and interfering in any way with being your highest and best self? If so, perform this exercise to offer and receive forgiveness and love.

1. Take a minute to hold yourself gently.

2. Close your eyes and "see" the people or landscapes standing in front of you as you close your eyes. Extend your intention to heal, to forgive, and to let go of any negative ties or old hurts.

3. Start with yourself. Be gentle yet protected as you open your heart to repair. Find the place where the apology starts in you, then offer it to them.

4. Ask for forgiveness. Then, listen with your inner ears as they receive it and offer it back to you. Hear their words and see their gestures, or hear their gestures and see their words. (Dreamscapes do not follow the rules of linear waking life.) This may take more than one try, especially if it is an old, long-standing wound.

5. Once you have said the words needed, unwrap or unwind anything that is still binding you together in an unhealthy way. Then, send the ancestor back to the light (or, if the person is still alive, into the light of today) with healing, forgiveness, and love.

Chapter Nine

Ruth's Story

My colleague Ruth had been haunted by two repetitive dreams for as long as I had known her. Over the course of several years, her first repeating dream theme had morphed into another, opposite theme: from silence to sailor-worthy swearing and yelling.

Ruth was the youngest of two sisters. Her mother suffered from clinical depression long before Ruth was born. During Ruth's childhood, her mother was in and out of the hospital, but medication and treatment options did not really touch her ongoing depression until Ruth was a young adult. As a result, Ruth experienced her mother as absent and vacant during childhood. Paradoxically, the passivity of her mother's depression felt intrusive in its cloying pervasiveness, and any attempts her mother made to be close felt intrusive as well.

Ruth remembers being furious at her mother when she was a child, well before she understood the nature of mental illness. Ruth's father instructed her to be good and quiet so as not to aggravate her mother. She began having explosive temper tantrums at the age of five. Once, when her mom tried to get physically close, Ruth grabbed a kitchen knife and told her to back off. This attempt at closeness was experienced by Ruth as unsafe and intrusive, since the inevitable flip side of being close to her mother was chronic abandonment when the depression returned. Luckily, when Ruth was a young adult, selective serotonin reuptake inhibitors (SSRIs) became available. (This class of antidepressants includes Prozac, Zoloft, etc.) SSRIs helped Ruth's mother tremendously, and the two had about ten good years together.

This history explains some of Ruth's difficulty speaking up for herself, as she was told to suppress her feelings, swallow them down, and not upset her mother all throughout childhood. Ruth's first recurring dream theme lasted for about five or six years. In these dreams, her mouth was blocked, filled with taffy, putty, or gum that she couldn't get out, or her tongue was too large and she couldn't talk. Ruth would pull and pull but couldn't clear her mouth to speak; she could only make sounds. Ruth was silenced by this gunk. Dream circle members had many ideas for removing, dissolving, swallowing, or getting help with the taffy stuff, but the dreams kept recurring. At some point, the connection was made that in waking life, Ruth had a hard time speaking up and advocating for herself. While she worked on this in therapy and made some progress in her dreams, the dream theme didn't really change in any meaningful way.

Then, after about six years of taffy dreams, Ruth experienced a shift in her dreams. In one of her last dreams in this series, Ruth swallowed a ball of yarn, and after pulling and pulling the thread, she finally got it all out. Following the thread is a common mythological and fairy-tale theme. One of the most well-known is the Greek myth of the Labyrinth and the Minotaur at the center. The hero of the story, Theseus, unwound a ball of thread as he navigated the Labyrinth. After slaying the Minotaur, Theseus followed the thread back to entrance of the Labyrinth and successfully escaped. The thread allowed him to navigate the twisted Labyrinth, slay a monster, and escape safely.

Around the time that Ruth experienced this dream shift, there was a shift in her waking life as well: Ruth was betrayed by an old friend, and she felt hurt and furious. She shared details in dream circle and expressed her rage as she told us the story. Notably, Ruth had no trouble expressing herself in dream circle—no taffy was blocking her mouth now! Around the same time, she reported feeling unappreciated and overworked by her new supervisor at her long-term job, and after much consideration, Ruth decided to retire early.

Shortly after these two events, Ruth came to dream circle and reported that her husband told her she had been screaming out loud in her sleep. Not just screaming, but yelling "Fuck you!" and "Get the fuck out of here!" to unseen and unknown dream characters who were intruding. "Get out of my mouth and out of my house!" she yelled to the intruders and the taffy.

Speaking up in her dreams and in waking life was a big change for Ruth. The outrageousness of her swearing gave her a great deal of mirth since it was so out of character. That was a piece of humor in the healing. As Ruth shared her pain and rage with the dream circle, we joined her in the enjoyment of her foul-mouthed dreaming self, and the power of healing community was evoked as well. Ruth then shared that her cousin and paternal grandmother also screamed while dreaming; it seemed to be a family pattern.

So, Ruth's recurrent dream themes morphed from the blocked-mouth themes to themes of intrusion and the need for protection. In her new series of dreams, Ruth's house was repeatedly invaded. As this theme continued, Ruth found herself defending her home more and more in her dreams, using various weapons and a very loud voice. Clearly something had shifted; Ruth was accessing anger and hurt that seemed deep and old, older than her current life circumstances.

Ruth shared that in her swearing dreams, she was still mad at her mother, and she felt intruded upon in the home invasion dreams. She was particularly concerned that she couldn't seem to let go of the anger, even though she understood the context now. This was something that we decided to work on.

I asked, "What do you need or want to hear from your parents?"

Ruth said, "I have forgiven them in my head, but I am still so mad. I feel it in my throat and chest and esophagus and voice. I still want to shout and get it out."

"You know, you had the right to feel angry. How old is the youngest part of you that feels so angry?"

"Really young, maybe four or five," Ruth said.

"Okay, let's get some protection for all the parts of you, including the youngest parts before we go on. What do you need right now to be safe from being and feeling invaded?"

Ruth answered, "A shield, like an old-fashioned one with full-body armor that has a strong logo on it. Maybe the logo says 'keep out!'"

I continued with the GAIA method. "Great. Put it on and hold your shield. Is that enough? Do you need anything else?"

"No, that's good."

"Does your little girl part feel shielded and protected too?"

"Yes, it is big enough for the adult me and for her too."

I continued, "Okay, can you now tell the angry girl part that it was normal and legitimate for her to feel this anger? Can she hear you, the adult you?"

"She sort of hears."

"And what happens then?"

"Not sure…" Ruth trailed off.

"That's okay, it's common not to know or be sure. So, let's take some deep breaths; we'll do it together." We paused to breathe. Then, I said, "Now, have the sixty-year-old part of you tell the angry little girl that she is all grown up; she even has a child of her own who is a teenager. Let her know that you can handle it. Tell her that she can turn it over to you. You already know how to be a good parent to your daughter and can parent this angry little girl part as well. When you and she are both ready, give her a hug and see what happens."

"When I hug her, she hugs back, and we become one. It's kind of like we melt into each other."

This melting hug is an ideal resolution in this kind of work, as the separated, hurt parts join with the competent adult self who has the resources, and they become one. When it doesn't happen this way, I help the dreamer along by encouraging the two parts to get closer and connect physically in some way, even if they are not quite ready to hug and unite.

There was also an intergenerational gift here: Ruth stopped the pattern. Her own daughter does not scream in the night and has never reported nightmares either; her ups and downs seem to have more to do with what is currently going on in her life rather than the past, typical for a teen.

A key takeaway from Ruth's story is that when we ask in dreamwork "And then what happens?" or "What happens next?" it is perfectly okay not to know. It is perfectly okay to say, "I don't know" until you do. You can also add the word *yet*—one of my favorite therapeutic words! "I don't know yet" keeps your options open and allows the potential of moving through the not knowing to a place of more knowing. You could also ask the dreamer something like, "If you did know, what would it be?" or "Is there a part of you that knows?" You may be surprised at their answer!

Spiral and Circle Healing

Like the Greek Labyrinth, spirals have a repeating pattern. Just as spirals occur spontaneously in nature (the fiddlehead fern, the nautilus shell, the sweep of the galaxies…), they occur in everyday life as well. Each time you move up the spiral of your timeline, you have a different and elevated perspective on what has occurred before, and you can use this new perspective to heal yourself, your lineage, and the planet. You will see things differently as you navigate the spiral.

In an ancient healing pilgrimage ritual in Jerusalem, both before and after the time that Jesus lived there, mourners and others who were suffering were invited to enter the temple space moving counterclockwise, and they were met by community members moving clockwise. As each sufferer passed by a community member, they received a warm gaze, a hug, or some words of kindness, then spiraled out again in the opposite direction.[79] This type of circling spiral concretizes and embodies the healing that can be found in connection and in community.

EXERCISE
Spiral Healing

When you have identified an ancestor who is still suffering and you think or know that this is still affecting you now, try this exercise.

1. When you are ready, surround yourself with the sapphire-blue container of light.

2. In your mind's eye, imagine a spiral shape going from the bottom to the top of the light container. Imagine your oldest-known ancestor's pain or trauma at the bottom of the spiral and your current time and place at the top.

3. Think about what happened to your ancestor in the context of the land they were living in and the time frame that it happened. Then, slowly move your consciousness up the spiral a ways, tracing the path in your mind's eye. Stop to rest and notice where you are. Notice the time frame and the context. What else do you see now that your vision has expanded? What else do you see from this higher, more distant perspective? What else rounds out the picture? Actively look for sources of comfort, healing, understanding, or compassion that you couldn't see

---

79. Brous, *The Amen Effect*.

when they were right in front of your face. By orienting your vision toward the positive, you can broaden your perspective. After all, we see what we are looking for.

4. Travel a few more rounds up the spiral, then stop and rest. What else do you see? What new understandings do you have? As you get more distance from your ancestor and travel up the spiral, can you sense the tug and the pull of the past lessening and loosening? With distance from the events, a wider worldview, and ascension toward the Divine, the pain lessens and healing takes hold.

5. When you have reached the top of the spiral and are back in the present moment, place a seal on this work, and know that you can extend the spiral onward as you learn more in this life.

Dream Functions to Help Heal and Grow

Working with your dreams gives you opportunity to heal yourself and your ancestors in real time. In your dreams, it is always now; it is never yesterday or tomorrow. So, if you are visited in dreamtime, by definition, it is present time. When you work with your dreams in waking life, you bring that sense of now into the present as well. It is the same for working with synchronicities that occur in everyday life.

David Leong writes that dreams are experiential realms that act as a sandbox for emotional regulation. Within the safety of the dream state, one can process and integrate emotional experiences without immediate real-world repercussions, allowing for a rehearsal that can aid in coping strategies and emotional resilience in waking life.[80] Dreams may also serve as a bridge between wakefulness and other states of consciousness, melding awareness and unconscious processes and allowing you to consider your experience of reality.

Dream expert Kelly Bulkeley articulates several of the many functions of dreaming.

---

80. Leong and Zinych, "Dreams as Portals to Parallel Realities and Reflections of Self."

Play: rooted in the evolutionary biology of play; a stimulus for flexibility, adaptability, and openness to novel experiences.

Healing: promoting recovery from illness and trauma; recognized by caregivers all over the world.

Artistic inspiration: artists don't simply use their dreams; some dreams use their artists.

Memory/learning: processing emotional experiences from the day and integrating them into one's ongoing sense of self.

Anticipatory: looking ahead to future possibilities, preparing for both dangers and opportunities.

Spiritual discovery: prompting heightened existential awareness; stimulating new religious beliefs throughout history.[81]

Read through this list again, and consider how each category might help in terms of ancestral healing and intergenerational wounds. Which of these many functions do you or your ancestors need from your dreams?

Humor and Healing

A key part of the healing process is humor. It is not a coincidence that humor often has its roots in trauma and heartache. Think of comedians you are familiar with and reflect on how much mileage they get out of breakups, health issues, stories about their children or parents, and dysfunctional family dynamics. Being able to laugh at yourself can salve the wound and allow you to move on. Thanks to neuropsychologist Donald Hebb, we know that neurons that fire together, wire together.[82] So, when you blend your memories of pain with humor, you create a new wiring, sometimes gentle, sometimes bawdy, sometimes raucous.

Here's an example of blending humor with ancestral work. My client Maria recalled the family tradition of cutting off the top of a ham before cooking it for Easter dinner. When her daughter asked her why she did this, Maria replied, "I don't know. That's the way I learned to do it from my

---

81. Bulkeley, "The Many Functions of Dreaming."
82. Krupic, "Wire Together, Fire Apart."

mother. Let's ask her." When they asked Maria's mother, she said, "That's what my mother taught me! Let's ask Nona." When they asked Maria's ninety-three-year-old grandmother why they needed to cut off the top of the ham before cooking it, she replied, "Are you still doing that? Bah! Back in the old country, my oven was too small, and it just didn't fit!" This family tradition was no longer necessary.

Each of us passes customs or habits to our descendants through parenting styles, wisdom, ideas, genetics, energy, and dreams or nightmares. How often do you catch yourself saying or doing something that reminds you of your parent or grandparent? You may make this discovery with delight or woe.

Art and Healing

My friend Mel, an artist, uses intuitive processes to create his art. At a recent art show, he shared that he stands before his blank canvases—three of them at a time—and listens to the canvases speak to him. He enters a waking dream state with his canvases, brushes, and paints, then "dances with one hand" to the music he hears and turns it into art.

Mel's abstract art often contains hints of early hieroglyphs that gradually morph into Hebrew letters. Black backgrounds, which may have a splash of a primary color on top, often contain a mysterious red or yellow circle. Mel shared that he didn't know why so many of his paintings had this element. Then, on a trip to Barcelona, a tour guide told Mel that before the Inquisition, Jews were forced to wear red or yellow circles on their clothes to identify themselves as Jewish. Mel's ancestors came from Spain; they were Sephardic Jews. Mel's ancestral legacy had made its way into his work. This time, rather than the red or yellow circle being used to shun and vilify, Mel uses the symbol for art and beauty. Memory, like art, can have a cascading effect.

A friend of mine, Janet, was cleaning out her parents' house after her mother's sudden death. She found many objects that she just couldn't dispose of, as they were all that Janet had left of her mother. Providentially, she came across a huge piece of corrugated cardboard. When she ripped a little of the facing off, it revealed a honeycomb of small compartments perfect for stowing things. Janet used the cardboard to make assemblage art, a type of artwork where each little piece of the assemblage evokes a memory and carries a story. Janet filled the cardboard honeycomb with bits of the flotsam and jetson of her parents' lives, as well as things she had collected: beach shells, plastic stars, acorn hats, little photos, a lobster claw, an old watch face, and more.

Janet's assemblage art became a weave of treasured items from her parents' lives, her own life, her children's lives, and the lives of others who had touched the family. Ultimately, it was an assemblage of family and community, a meditation on things left behind that conjure up memories. Remnants of other times, places, and people.

Compassionate conversations with your ancestors can be filled with creativity, love, and invitation. You can dance their stories, write poems or songs about their sagas, make art, or even write a play. Take old photos and make an ancestor gallery along your staircase. Write down the details of your dream visits. Notice synchronicities when they show up in your waking life, and honor and share them.

The therapeutic modality Internal Family Systems proposes that when an individual is functioning as their highest and most integrated self—not fragmented parts that take over or hijack their wholeness—they embrace the eight c's: compassion, curiosity, courage, calm, clarity, confidence, creativity, and connectedness. It is not a coincidence that many of these qualities have been highlighted in this chapter and throughout the book. Be in relationship with the living and the dead while maintaining good and healthy boundaries. Have the centeredness to bring caring and commemoration (three more c's!) into these relationships. This will heal your fragmented self, restore family ties, and allow your unmourned ancestors to take their place on the family tree.

TEN

HOW TO BECOME A WISE AND GOOD FUTURE ANCESTOR

> Trauma resolved is a blessing of great power.
> —*Peter Levine,* Waking the Tiger

There are many paths to recognizing, honoring, healing, and setting good boundaries with your ancestors—it is a lifelong journey. Your life began millennia ago, and your legacy will continue in perpetuity whether or not you have children and grandchildren of your own. Those whose lives you touch—as a family member, auntie or uncle, teacher, mentor, neighbor, artist, or writer, to name a few—become part of your chosen or affiliated family, your down-line. Your actions and words take on a life of their own, so pay attention to the acts of support and kindness you can add to the world bank. It is good to attend to this when you think about what kind of ancestor you want to be. Repairs and blessings are always available.

The two keywords and actions that honor and heal your ties with your ancestors are *relationship* and *connection*. During the last several years, many people have been writing about the epidemic of loneliness that has engulfed modern society. COVID-19 was a big hit, and the fallout from shifting to a preponderance of online work and socialization rather than being in-person has made it worse. Add to that social media, smartphones, violence in the streets, and political unrest, and we have a society of lonely and disconnected people—unless we take conscious steps to rectify this.

Each of us desperately needs to reconnect with the living and with encounters in waking life to thrive. You can amplify and strengthen your life when you actively connect with your ancestors and your dreams as well. Both your dreams and your ancestors can give you tips, hints, and advice about how to bring more joy and connection to waking life. Each of us needs to recount and remember for both the dead and the living.

Ancestral trauma can be passed down for generations, but as you learned in this book, once you break the cycle of silence, you open the world of choice to yourself and future generations. If people can inherit wounds, they can also inherit resilience, strength, and connections. The experiences and dreams in this book provided context to help you understand from the inside and the outside.

The six types of calls you may get from your ancestors serve as a structure and guide to your work with the departed. There are ancestors to simply honor and connect with, and there are those who offer you gifts or blessings as well as those who need help in a variety of ways. All of them have the same request: for you to remember them, to teach their stories to your descendants so that their lives will not have been in vain and their teachings will live on.

The theme of bones was woven throughout this book: literal bones, metaphorical bones, and what the marrow of your bones means for you and your lineage. Marrow is the lifeblood inside your bones that can quite literally heal. This is where stem cells come from. Epigenetics and inherited traits and patterns in your life encompass the nature/nurture side of inheritance. These patterns get passed down through the generations, showing up as lived experiences or strong dream memories for great-grandchildren.

How you heal, the stages of grief, complicated grief, and your role with departed ancestors are key. The continuum of consciousness gave perspective on deeper connections with the departed than you may have thought possible. Removing your loved ones from a crypt of silence allows you to fully grieve and honor them.

Your body is the home of your soul, your thoughts, and your emotions. Intergenerational trauma can show up in all these arenas and in the embodied nature of intergenerational trauma transmission.

Connections Heal

Connections heal, no matter when or how we get them, including finding your Wise Elder from beyond the veil to guide and support you. The science and philosophy of timelessness help us to expand your reach and repertoire. And in this chapter, you begin your final ascent into becoming a future great ancestor yourself.

Wise ancestors can come in many forms. I have run into several former students from my days as a professor at Boston University School of Social Work. It has been about sixteen years since I taught there, so I don't always recognize former students when they approach me, but as soon as they identify themselves, I do. I am always honored and tickled that they remember me as a mentor who affected their life and professional choices. Some of them are now professors themselves! When former students tell me that they are still teaching my relational model of group development in their classes, it feels like my legacy, and I am delighted. Another form of passing on ancestral wisdom.

Legacies Etched Deeply

When a loved one's bones are buried in a specific location, it can make a place sacred. There is something powerful about having a place to visit, though it's not an option for every family nor desired by all. Sometimes the choice is not available because of war or natural disasters. Sometimes cremation is the right choice to honor your ancestors' wishes. Sometimes loved ones wish for their ashes to be scattered. Even if there is not an exact place you can visit a loved one, make note of where you poured their ashes or you would have buried them, had you been able to—this then becomes sacred ground for you and your family.

My family has a little cat cemetery in our backyard. Each time one of our beloved kitties passes, we bury them behind the forsythia in a protected alcove with a stone commemorating the grave. Our cat Effie's twin brother died last year. Effie escaped the house recently, and one of the first things he did was run out to the backyard and nose around the spot his brother was buried. How did he know?

There is something powerful about having a special spot to connect to loved ones for all eternity. My friend Jules spent some quality time with her ancestors at their gravesite. She knew their history and viscerally felt the sorrow and pain of their lives as she sat with them there. As a deeply spiritual being, Jules was moved to offer a healing prayer. She added personal prayers for each family member. At some point, she had a felt sense of the sadness lifting and felt content. She has continued to pray for her ancestors' healing.

EXERCISE
Ancestral Meditation

To reflect on your journey to your ancestors and to honor them, learn from them, and take their teachings into your life going forward, try this guided meditation created by Diane Pardes. Take a moment to prepare to connect with your ancestors, to connect with the ones who have nurtured your spirit and your life, and to receive their blessings and gifts. You might decide to record yourself reading through the meditation and then play it back so that you can immerse yourself fully in the imagery.

1. Get into a comfortable position. Relax your forehead, jaw, eyes, and shoulders. Focus inward. Take several slow, deep breaths.

2. When you are ready, begin the meditation.

    Picture yourself walking toward a cave where your ancestors are buried. Slowly you descend the steps, pausing at each level. You enter the cave opening, surrounded by womb-like, protective walls.

    As you descend further, you reach an opening leading to a double chamber of caves. Its walls hold the wisdom of your ancestors, who have been through so much yet persevered. You can feel their presence. They lead the way for you now and are always there when you need them.

    Think about the special ones who had a major impact on your life—who knew and loved you when embodied as liv-

ing, breathing souls. What wisdom have they taught you? What are they trying to share with you right now? Feel it and take it all in. Take a few moments to rest here.

Before you leave, honor them for their gifts and lessons and for paving the path forward.

It is now time to return, taking the treasures, teachings, and wisdom from your ancestors back to the land of the living, and to incorporate them into your life.

Begin retracing your footsteps, slowly emerging from the womb-like cave. Think about what you have experienced and learned as you carry it forward into the sunlight.

3. After you have completed the meditation, take some time to write down what you have learned and discovered. Pay attention to this, as it is a guide to inform your life's purpose and meaning.

★ ★ ★

It is not only humans that have memories; plants and trees carry memory traces as well. We know that trees are connected underground through an interlaced fungal structure known as mycorrhizal networks, or the "wood-wide web." This might be their ancestral connection system. Older trees are known as "mother trees" and share nutrients with their seedlings to help them survive.[83] Trees act to protect their next generation. We, too, can act to protect the next generation.

Checklist for Becoming a Good Ancestor

Angeline Boulley writes, "People say to think seven generations ahead when making big life decisions, because our future ancestors—those yet to arrive, who will one day become the Elders—live with the choices we make today."[84] While this is not a complete list of everything you can do to

---

83. Grant, "Do Trees Talk to Each Other?"
84. Boulley, *Firekeeper's Daughter*, 237.

become a Wise Elder, it is a good start. See how many of these actions you are already taking and note what else you may be called to do.

- Tell the stories of your ancestors, your non-biological ancestors, and your ancestral lands. Your non-biological ancestors may include teachers, mentors, or spiritual leaders. Your ancestral lands include where you live now, the lands your ancestors came from, and lands that are holy to you, whether your ancestors lived on them physically or held them sacred in their traditions.
- Teach and share these stories and legacies with your children and your children's children, your nieces and nephews, and your non-biological descendants, including your students, clients (if appropriate), and colleagues.
- Make a genogram and update it periodically as new members of the family are born, die, marry in, or have some change in status. Recently, I had to do this myself when a family member asked to see the family genogram and I realized I was overdue for an update by many years: some new babies, a few deaths, and a recent marriage.
- Are there gaps in your family tree because someone who died was never talked about, such as a child who died young or a member who took their own life? See if someone can tell you their story—not only of who they were and how they died, but of their life and how they lived as well. This way, they become a part of you, your life, and your history. Who still knows their story? Listen to the spaces in the stories and the silences; here you may find the answers.
- In addition to oral storytelling and sharing, write things down. Keep a journal, write a poem or a short story or a play, or use the base of your ancestors' lives as the scaffolding for historical fiction, as so many writers are doing today. In Amy Harmon's book *What the Wind Knows*, a grandfather tells his granddaughter that if she can't speak the words, to write them down. Writing them gives them somewhere to go.
- Make the foods your ancestors prepared. Ask your parents or grandparents for the recipe—even better if you can get a copy of it in their own handwriting! Let the recipients of these foods know where they

came from. At Thanksgiving, for example, say, "This is Grandma Edie's stuffing recipe."

- In your garden, plant the flowers they would have planted. I remember the gladiolas in both my grandma Molly's yard and my parents'. I thought of them when I had my first real garden as an adult with my own home. Harvest the teachings and the crops of your ancestors. Tend the literal and metaphorical fields of their plantings in your garden or your mind.
- Wear their jewelry and talismans, and tell the stories of each piece. Feel your ancestor with you when you do this. Tell the story of how the item came to them, if you know it. Was it an heirloom or a gift from a special occasion? Share that too.
- Learn a craft that they knew, such as knitting or wood carving or cross-stitch. Is there a pattern or a style that they loved that you could embrace? Were they fond of a particular color or image? Use that.
- Build and create your shrines. Donate a plaque to your place of worship, or dedicate a bench overlooking their favorite spot in the park in their name and honor. These shrines then become thresholds in time and space. For example, my neighbor (my daughter's honorary auntie Innes) used to volunteer at the local elementary school, and there is a bench with her name on it next to the playground where the children still swing and run and slide.
- Show up. At my brother-in-law Jim's memorial service, he was remembered fondly as a good friend and neighbor who showed up with a shovel or snowplow to help others dig themselves out during the snowy Buffalo winters. Show up for others like Jim.
- Remember and commemorate the anniversary of an ancestor's birth and their death. Light a votive or yahrzeit candle and say a prayer out loud or to yourself. May their memories be for a blessing. May you be for a blessing. May all your descendants be for a blessing.

Maria Popover writes, "It may be that we evolved to dream ourselves into reality."[85] A laboratory of consciousness exists where the never-never land between waking consciousness and the unconsciousness of sleep is the practice ground of impossibility, where the impossible becomes possible. Where not only our hopes and prayers are with our ancestors and descendants, but where our very best dreams become manifest.

May my blessings join with yours for our future generations. May we all be healed and made whole backward and forward in time and space. And may it be so.

---

85. Popova, "What Birds Dream About."

ACKNOWLEDGMENTS

This book has been a seed in my heart and mind for several years. A few years ago, I had a dream, to quote Dr. King, that clearly connected me with some of my ancestors in a way that had never happened to me before. Not only did I have a dream about borscht, the beet soup my Ukrainian great-grandparents probably ate, but I had a synchronistic overlap of becoming a small part of contributing to healing from the ravages of war in the Ukraine with my previous book, *PTSDreams*. An American aid volunteer there, Jose Lara, came across my book *PTSDreams* and began using it to help the Ukrainians with their nightmares from war trauma. I felt honored to be of assistance. My work was being shared in the land of my ancestors. Clearly, it was time for this next book to be born.

I am so appreciative of all my friends, family, clients, and colleagues that contributed to this book. When I let it be known that I was collecting stories and experiences of ancestor dreaming and ancestral encounters and experiences of all kinds, I received a robust response. Some people sent me one dream; others sent me an enormous packet of both their sleeping dreams and their waking experiences with the departed that they had been collecting for years—or decades, or generations. Some really wanted their own names to be used; it was important for them to finally be named out loud and publicly. Others were willing to use their names, and some preferred to have their stories told by pseudonym. All the dreams and stories have been vetted with the contributor to assure integrity of reporting, and personal details have been altered to further protect privacy. I give a special thanks to my family, who allowed me to publicly share pieces of our family

Acknowledgments

story, and in the process of doing so, many of us became closer and forged new connections. Thanks go to my brothers David and Bobby Schiller and Bob Krohn, my sisters Debbie and Lynnie Krohn, my nieces, and especially to my husband Steve and our daughter Sara, who have generously been both sharers and readers.

Thank you to my wonderful personal dream circle of over forty years, Lisa Kennedy and Marcia Lewin-Berlin, my longest sister/friend, Diane Pardes, for her endless support of my writing and my life, my sister/friends Julie Leavitt, Beth Rontal, Sara Levine, and my circle of Torah study women with whom I have been studying weekly for over thirty years. And to my professional dream circle who have become my friends as well, Mia Woodruff, Joy Weider, Joyce Friedman, Ruth Silverstein, Ellen Kruger, and members emeritus Starr Potts and Marcia Post. And as always, thanks to Eve Diana who started me on the dreaming path to my life's work these many years ago.

The organization IASD, the International Association for the Study of Dreams, has become part of my family over the past fifteen years. I have been stimulated, excited, awed, and supported by this group. They have published my articles in their journal *DreamTime*, reviewed my previous books, interviewed me on podcasts and radio, and provided me with a worldwide posse of dear friends and dreamers. Special callout to David Kahn, who introduced me to this organization, creating another overlap in our circles of dance, spirituality, and now dream life, and dear dream friends Marta Aarli, Katherine Bell, Jean Campbell, Jason DeBord, Tzivia Gover, Bob Hoss, Claire Johnson, Kim Mascaro, Victoria Rabinow, and Lauren Schneider.

Many thanks go to Llewellyn Worldwide for their support and encouragement of my writing over the years, and for making it so easy to get this book started! Big appreciation to Amy Glaser, acquisitions editor, for seeing my potential, to Nicole Borneman for making the book tighter and more coherent with her editorial skills, and to Kat Neff for her excellent marketing support.

Acknowledgments

Finally, a deep appreciation to all my ancestors who came before me and guided my heart and hands to share their experiences and connect, across time and space, with others who also had ancestors needing to be remembered and stories needing to be told. This is for you.

BIBLIOGRAPHY

"About AEDP Psychotherapy." AEDP Institute. Accessed January 14, 2025. https://aedpinstitute.org/about-aedp/.

Adler, Benjamin. "Introduction to Kabbalah: The Creation Myth." Sefaria. Accessed May 1, 2025. https://www.sefaria.org/sheets/32246.

Anisfeld, Sharon Cohen. "A Blessing from Jerusalem for the Month of Shevat." Hebrew College, January 11, 2024. https://hebrewcollege.edu/blog/a-blessing-from-jerusalem-for-the-month-of-shevat/.

"Anishinabe Dreams." Native American Netroots, September 25, 2010. http://nativeamericannetroots.net/diary/691.

Arendt, Hannah. *The Human Condition*. 2nd ed. University of Chicago Press, 2018.

Ayao, Edward Halealoha. "Native Burials: Human Rights and Sacred Bones." *Cultural Survival Quarterly* 24, no. 1 (2010). https://www.culturalsurvival.org/publications/cultural-survival-quarterly/native-burials-human-rights-and-sacred-bones.

Baldwin, Michael, and Deborah Korn. *Every Memory Deserves Respect: EMDR, the Proven Trauma Therapy with the Power to Heal*. Workman Publishing, 2021.

"Bones Chapel in Evora, Sao Francisco Church." Visit Evora. Accessed April 29, 2025. https://www.visitevora.net/en/bones-chapel-evora/.

Boulley, Angeline. *Firekeeper's Daughter*. Square Fish, 2021.

Brach, Tara. "De-Conditioning the Hungry Ghosts." Psychology Today, September 5, 2017. https://www.psychologytoday.com/us/blog/finding-true-refuge/201709/de-conditioning-the-hungry-ghosts.

Brewster, Fanny. *Race and the Unconscious: An Africanist Depth Psychology Perspective on Dreaming*. Routledge, 2023.

Brous, Sharon. *The Amen Effect: Ancient Wisdom to Mend Our Broken Hearts and World*. Avery, 2024.

Bulkeley, Kelly. "The Many Functions of Dreaming." Psychology Today, June 28, 2023. https://www.psychologytoday.com/us/blog/dreaming-in-the-digital-age/202306/the-many-functions-of-dreaming.

Bynum, Edward Bruce. "The African Origin of Familial Consciousness and the Dynamics of Dreaming." *Dreaming* 31, no. 2 (2021): 91–99. https://www.doi.org/10.1037/drm0000171.

Casale, Alessandro. "Indigenous Dreams." Indigenous New Hampshire Collaborative Collective, January 25, 2019. https://indigenousnh.com/2019/01/25/indigenous-dreams/.

Chishti. "Sufism and Dreams." The Sufi Tavern, February 15, 2018. https://sufi-tavern.com/sufi-doctrine/sufism-and-dreams/.

Cooke, Michael. "DOE Explains…the Higgs Bosun." US Department of Energy. Accessed January 9, 2025. https://www.energy.gov/science/doe-explainsthe-higgs-boson.

Cronkleton, Emily. "What Is Holotropic Breathwork and How Is It Used?" Healthline. Updated September 18, 2018. https://www.healthline.com/health/holotropic-breathwork.

Dana, Deb. *The Polyvagal Theory in Therapy: Engaging the Rhythm of Regulation*. W. W. Norton, 2018.

Dannu, Ayala. "Ancestral Dreaming and Why It Needs to Be a Part of the Dream Studies Conversation." *DreamTime Magazine* 36, no. 3 (Sept. 2019): 12–13.

Dunlea, Marian. *BodyDreaming in the Treatment of Developmental Trauma: An Embodied Therapeutic Approach*. Routledge, 2019.

"Early Hawaiians." National Park Service. Updated June 8, 2021. https://www.nps.gov/hale/learn/historyculture/early-hawaiians.htm.

Easter, Sandra. *Jung and the Ancestors: Beyond Biography, Mending the Ancestral Web*. Aeon Books, 2015.

Eickelkamp, Ute. "Sand Storytelling: Its Social Meaning in Anangu Children's Lives." In *Growing up in Central Australia: New Anthropological Studies of Aboriginal Childhood and Adolescence*, edited by Ute Eickelkamp, 109–30. Berghahn Books, 2011.

Ellis, Leslie. *A Clinician's Guide to Dream Therapy: Implementing Simple and Effective Dreamwork*. Routledge, 2019.

Ellis, Leslie. "Dreams of Bereavement: How Your Dreams Help You Grieve." Dr. Leslie Ellis, October 25, 2020. https://drleslieellis.com/how-your-dreams-help-you-grieve-2/.

Faust, Jamy, and Peter Faust. *The Constellation Approach: Finding Peace Through Your Family Lineage*. Regent Press, 2015.

Firestone, Tirzah. *Wounds into Wisdom: Healing Intergenerational Jewish Trauma*. Monkfish Book Publishing Company, 2019.

Forbes, Jack D. "Indigenous Americans: Spirituality and Ecos." *Dædalus* 130, no. 4 (Fall 2001): 283–300.

Ford, Jamie. *The Many Daughters of Afong Moy*. Atria Books, 2022.

Fosha, Diana. "'Nothing that Feels Bad Is Ever the Last Step': The Role of Positive Emotions in Experiential Work with Difficult Emotional Experiences." *Clinical Psychology & Psychotherapy* 11, no. 1 (Jan./Feb. 2004): 30–43. https://doi.org/10.1002/cpp.390.

Fosha, Diana. "Wired for Healing: Thirteen Ways of Looking at AEDP." AEDP Institute. Accessed April 22, 2025. https://aedpinstitute.org/journal/wired-for-healing/.

Frankl, Viktor E. *Man's Search for Meaning*. Beacon Press, 2006.

García, Jordi Borràs. "Dreams for a Collective Crisis." *DreamTime Magazine* (Winter 2019): 21–23. https://www.academia.edu/38243293/Dreams_for_a_Collective_Crisis.

Gendlin, Eugene T. *Focusing*. Bantam, 1982.

Gendlin, Eugene T. *Let Your Body Interpret Your Dreams*. Chiron Publications, 1986.

Bibliography

Glaskin, Katie. "Dreams, Perception, and Creative Realization." *Topics in Cognitive Science* 7, no. 4 (Oct. 2015): 664–76. https://doi.org/10.1111/tops.12157.

Grant, Richard. "Do Trees Talk to Each Other?" *Smithsonian Magazine*, March 2018. https://www.smithsonianmag.com/science-nature/the-whispering-trees-180968084/.

Harjo, Joy. *Poet Warrior: A Memoir.* W. W. Norton, 2021.

Harmon, Amy. *What the Wind Knows.* Lake Union Publishing, 2019.

Henriques, Martha. "Can the Legacy of Trauma Be Passed Down the Generations?" BBC, March 26, 2019. https://www.bbc.com/future/article/20190326-what-is-epigenetics.

Herman, Judith. *Trauma and Recovery: The Aftermath of Violence—From Domestic Abuse to Political Terror.* Basic Books, 1992.

"How to Help Your Clients Understand Their Window of Tolerance." National Institute for the Clinical Application of Behavioral Medicine. Accessed April 29, 2025. https://www.nicabm.com/trauma-how-to-help-your-clients-understand-their-window-of-tolerance/.

Hübl, Thomas. *Healing Collective Trauma: A Process for Integrating Our Intergenerational and Cultural Wounds.* Sounds True, 2020.

Hughes, Daniel A. *Building the Bonds of Attachment: Awakening Love in Deeply Troubled Children.* Jason Aronson, 2000.

"Introduction." Florida State University Chemistry & Biochemistry. Accessed January 14, 2025. https://www.chem.fsu.edu/chemlab/chm1045lmanual/conserve/introduction.html.

Johnson, Clare R. *The Art of Transforming Nightmares: Harness the Creative and Healing Power of Bad Dreams, Sleep Paralysis, and Recurring Nightmares.* Llewellyn Publications, 2021.

Johnson, Clare R. *Llewellyn's Complete Book of Lucid Dreaming: A Comprehensive Guide to Promote Creativity, Overcome Sleep Disturbances & Enhance Health and Wellness.* Llewellyn Publications, 2017.

Johnson, Myke. "Broken Shards of Light." *Finding Our Way Home* (blog), November 16, 2013. https://findingourwayhome.blog/2013/11/16/broken-shards-of-light.

Jung, C. G. *Memories, Dreams, Reflections*. Reissue. Edited by Aniela Jaffé. Translated by Richard Winston and Clara Winston. Vintage Books, 1965.

Jung, C. G. *The Red Book: A Reader's Edition*. Edited by Sonu Shamdasani. Translated by Sonu Shamdasani, John Peck, and Mark Kyburz. W. W. Norton, 2009.

Kaehr, Shelley A. *Heal Your Ancestors to Heal Your Life: The Transformative Power of Genealogical Regression*. Llewellyn Publications, 2022.

Keller, Irwin. "In These Last Months of 2023, I Have Noticed the Jewish Ancestors in Me More than Ever." Jewish Telegraphic Agency, December 29, 2023. https://www.jta.org/2023/12/29/ideas/in-these-last-months-i-have-noticed-the-jewish-ancestors-in-me-more-than-ever.

Kellermann, Natan P. F. "Epigenetic Transmission of Holocaust Trauma: Can Nightmares Be Inherited?" *Israel Journal of Psychiatry and Related Sciences* 50, no. 1 (Sept. 2013).

Kingsford-Smith, Andrew. "Disguised in Dance: The Secret History of Capoeira." Culture Trip, July 7, 2021. https://theculturetrip.com/south-america/brazil/articles/disguised-in-dance-the-secret-history-of-capoeira.

Krenak, Ailton. *Ideas to Postpone the End of the World*. Anansi International, 2020.

Krippner, Stanley. Foreword to *Modern Psychology and Ancient Wisdom: Psychological Healing Practices from the World's Religious Traditions*, 2nd ed., by Sharon G. Mijares. Routledge, 2016.

Krippner, Stanley, and April Thompson. "A 10-Facet Model of Dreaming Applied to Dream Practices of Sixteen Native American Cultural Groups." *Dreaming* 6, no. 2 (1996): 71–96.

Krupic, Julija. "Wire Together, Fire Apart." *Science* 357, no. 6355 (2017). https://doi.org/10.1126/science.aao4159.

"Kübler-Ross Change Curve." Elisabeth Kübler-Ross Foundation. Accessed February 18, 2025. https://www.ekrfoundation.org/5-stages-of-grief/change-curve/.

Kübler-Ross, Elisabeth. *On Death and Dying*. Scribner, 2011.

Leong, David P. *Street Signs: Toward a Missional Theology of Urban Cultural Engagement*. Pickwick Publications, 2012.

Leong, David, and Oxana Zinych. "Dreams as Portals to Parallel Realities and Reflections of Self." Qeios, December 18, 2023. https://doi.org/10.32388/242XCF.

Levine, Peter A. *Healing Trauma: A Pioneering Program for Restoring the Wisdom of Your Body*. Sounds True, 2008.

Levine, Peter A., and Ann Frederick. *Waking the Tiger: Healing Trauma*. North Atlantic Books, 1997.

Levy, Yael. *Directing the Heart: Weekly Mindfulness Teachings and Practices from the Torah*. A Way In, 2019.

Lipton, Bruce H. *The Biology of Belief: Unleashing the Power of Consciousness, Matter & Miracles*. 10th anniversary ed. Hay House, 2015.

Lipton, Bruce H. *The Wisdom of Your Cells: How Your Beliefs Control Your Biology*. Narrated by the author. Sounds True Audio, 2006. 8 hr., 8 min.

Marble, Mike. *How to Have a Good Life After You're Dead: Explorations into the Afterlife*. Oxford Book Writers, 2023.

Marks, Isaac. "Rehearsal Relief of a Nightmare." *The British Journal of Psychiatry* 33, no. 5 (Nov. 1978): 461–65. https://doi.org/10.1192/bjp.133.5.461.

Mascaro, Kimberly R. *Dream Medicine: The Intersection of Wellness and Consciousness*. McFarland, 2021.

Maté, Gabor. *When the Body Says No: Exploring the Stress-Disease Connection*. Trade Paper Press, 2011.

Maté, Gabor, and Daniel Maté. *The Myth of Normal: Trauma, Illness, and Healing in a Toxic Culture*. Vermillion, 2022.

Bibliography

Mayo Clinic Staff. "Stem Cells: What They Are and What They Do." Mayo Clinic, March 23, 2024. https://www.mayoclinic.org/tests-procedures/bone-marrow-transplant/in-depth/stem-cells/art-20048117.

Menakem, Resmaa. *My Grandmother's Hands: Racialized Trauma and the Pathway to Mending Our Hearts and Bodies.* Central Recovery Press, 2017.

Mindell, Arnold. *Dreambody: The Body's Role in Revealing the Self.* 2nd ed. Lao Tse Press, 1998.

Mindstar Health. "7 Native American Beliefs About Dreams that Open a Portal to the Other World." LinkedIn, May 16, 2023. https://www.linkedin.com/pulse/7-native-american-beliefs-dreams-open-portal-other-world/.

Moss, Robert. "Dreaming with the Departed." *The Robert Moss Blog*, April 30, 2020. https://mossdreams.blogspot.com/2017/04/dreaming-with-departed.html.

Moss, Robert. "Our Ancestors Are Looking for Us..." AZquotes. Accessed April 29, 2025. https://www.azquotes.com/quote/1490166.

Nakra, Rishabh. "How LHC Can Be the First Time Machine." The Secrets of the Universe. Accessed January 14, 2025. https://www.secretsofuniverse.in/first-time-machine-the-lhc/.

Nimoy, Leonard. "How Leonard Nimoy's Jewish Roots Inspired the Vulcan Salute." Star Trek, July 17, 2021. https://www.startrek.com/news/the-jewish-ritual-that-led-nimoy-to-create-the-vulcan-salute.

Nurick, Jennifer. "What Is the Window of Tolerance?" Psychotherapy Central, September 21, 2020. https://jennynurick.com/what-is-the-window-of-tolerance/.

Obama, Barack. *Dreams from My Father: A Story of Race and Inheritance.* Crown, 2004.

Obama, Michelle. *The Light We Carry: Overcoming in Uncertain Times.* Crown, 2024.

O'Donohue, John. *Beauty: The Invisible Embrace.* Harper Perennial, 2005.

Ogden, Pat, and Janina Fischer. *Sensorimotor Psychotherapy: Interventions for Trauma and Attachment*. W. W. Norton, 2019.

Ohlheiser, Abby. "The Jewish Roots of Leonard Nimoy and 'Live Long and Prosper.'" *The Washington Post*, February 27, 2015. https://www.washingtonpost.com/news/arts-and-entertainment/wp/2015/02/27/the-jewish-roots-of-leonard-nimoy-and-live-long-and-prosper/.

Oliver, Mary. *Upstream: Selected Essays*. Penguin Books, 2019.

Patton, Kimberley. "Dream Incubation: Theology and Topography." *DreamTime Magazine* 19, no. 4 (2002).

Popova, Maria. "What Birds Dream About: The Evolution of REM and How We Practice the Possible in Our Sleep." The Marginalian. Accessed January 9, 2025. https://www.themarginalian.org/2024/07/02/birds-dream-rem/.

Porges, Stephen W., and Deb Dana, eds. *Clinical Applications of Polyvagal Theory: The Emergence of Polyvagal-Informed Therapies*. W. W. Norton, 2018.

Porges, Stephen W., and Gregory F. Lewis. "The Polyvagal Hypothesis: Common Mechanisms Mediating Autonomic Regulation, Vocalizations, and Listening." *Handbook of Behavioral Neuroscience* 19 (2010): 255–64. https://doi.org/10.1016/B978-0-12-374593-4.00025-5.

Prechtel, Martín. *The Smell of Rain on Dust: Grief and Praise*. North Atlantic Books, 2015.

Price, Tiffany E. "Sherman Alexie's Reservation Blues: The Native American Journey Reflected in Dreams." *The Journal of South Texas English Studies* 6, no. 2 (Fall 2016): 47–55. https://scholarworks.utrgv.edu/cgi/viewcontent.cgi?article=1055&context=jostes.

"Rachel Yehuda, PhD." Mount Sinai. Accessed January 14, 2025. https://profiles.mountsinai.org/rachel-yehuda.

Rinpoche, Sogyal. *The Tibetan Book of Living and Dying: The Spiritual Classic and International Bestseller*. Rev. ed. Edited by Patrick D. Gaffney and Andrew Harvey. HarperOne, 2009.

Ríos, Alberto. "A House Called Tomorrow." Poets.org. Accessed February 11, 2025. https://poets.org/poem/house-called-tomorrow.

Bibliography

Rossner, Rena. *The Light of the Midnight Stars*. Hachette, 2021.

Rothschild, Babette. *The Body Remembers: The Psychophysiology of Trauma and Trauma Treatment*. W. W. Norton, 2010.

Rothschild, Babette. *8 Keys to Safe Trauma Recovery: Take-Charge Strategies to Empower Your Healing*. W. W. Norton, 2010.

Rubinstein, Tanya Taylor, ed. *Writing at Time's Edge*. Robb Thomson, 2014.

Schiller, Linda Yael. *Modern Dreamwork: New Tools for Decoding Your Soul's Wisdom*. Llewellyn Publications, 2019.

Schiller, Linda Yael. "Moving Into Your Dreams: Embracing Embodied Dreamwork." *DreamTime Magazine* (2020).

Schiller, Linda Yael. *PTSDreams: Transform Your Nightmares from Trauma through Healing Dreamwork*. Llewellyn Publications, 2022.

Schützenberger, Anne Ancelin. *The Ancestor Syndrome: Transgenerational Psychotherapy and the Hidden Links in the Family Tree*. Routledge, 2009.

Schwartz, Arielle. *The Post-Traumatic Growth Guidebook: Practical Mind-Body Tools to Heal Trauma, Foster Resilience, and Awaken Your Potential*. PESI Publishing & Media, 2020.

Schwartz, Richard. *Introduction to Internal Family Systems*. 2nd ed. Sounds True, 2023.

Shafak, Elif. *The Forty Rules of Love*. Penguin Books, 2010.

Shafak, Elif. *The Island of Missing Trees*. Bloomsbury Publishing, 2021.

Shainberg, Catherine. *Kabbalah and the Power of Dreaming: Awakening the Visionary Life*. Inner Traditions, 2005.

Shainberg, Catherine. *The Kabbalah of Light: Ancient Practices to Ignite the Imagination and Illuminate the Soul*. Inner Traditions, 2022.

Siegel, Daniel J. "Dr. Dan Siegal Explains 'Top Down' Constraints." PsychAlive, March 3, 2011. 3 min., 23 sec. https://www.youtube.com/watch?v=1rDumctR920.

Siegel, Daniel J. *The Mindful Brain: Reflection and Attunement in the Cultivation of Well-Being*. W. W. Norton, 2007.

Somé, Malidoma Patrice. *Ritual: Power, Healing, and Community*. Penguin Books, 1997.

"Songlines." Deadly Story. Accessed January 9, 2025. https://deadlystory.com/page/culture/Life_Lore/Songlines.

Swaim, Emily. "Imagery Rehearsal Therapy Can Help You Rewrite Nightmares for Sweeter Sleep." Healthline, August 19, 2022. https://www.healthline.com/health/sleep/imagery-rehearsal-therapy.

Taleb, Nassim Nicholas. *Antifragile: Things That Gain from Disorder*. Random House, 2014.

Tedlock, Barbara. "The Poetics and Spirituality of Dreaming: A Native American Enactive Theory." *Dreaming* 14, no. 2–3 (2004): 183–89. https://doi.org/10.1037/1053-0797.14.2-3.183.

Tevington, Patricia, and Manolo Corichi. "Many Americans Report Interacting with Dead Relatives in Dreams or Other Ways." Pew Research Center, August 23, 2023. https://www.pewresearch.org/short-reads/2023/08/23/many-americans-report-interacting-with-dead-relatives-in-dreams-or-other-ways/.

Thakurdas, Amy. "Ho'oponopono: Universal Healing Method for Mankind." *The International Journal of Healing and Caring* 8, no. 3 (Sept. 2008): https://irp-cdn.multiscreensite.com/891f98f6/files/uploaded/Thakurdas-8-3.pdf.

Tonkinson, Robert. *The Mardudjara Aborigines: Living the Dream in Australia's Desert*. Harcourt School, 1979.

Valeii, Kathi. "How Does Intergenerational Trauma Work?" Verywell Health. Updated December 5, 2024. https://www.verywellhealth.com/intergenerational-trauma-5191638.

Van der Kolk, Bessel. *The Body Keeps the Score: Brain, Mind, and Body in the Healing of Trauma*. Viking Press, 2018.

Volkan, Vamik D. *A Nazi Legacy: Depositing, Transgenerational Transmission, Dissociation, and Remembering Through Action*. Routledge, 2019.

Waggoner, Robert. *Lucid Dreaming: Gateway to the Inner Self*. Moment Point Press, 2009.

Wapner, Jessica. "The Paradox of Listening to Our Bodies." *The New Yorker*, July 6, 2023. https://www.newyorker.com/science/elements/the-paradox-of-listening-to-our-bodies.

"What Are Stem Cells?" University of Rochester Medical Center. Accessed January 14, 2025. https://www.urmc.rochester.edu/encyclopedia/content.aspx?contenttypeid=160&contentid=38.

Whyte, David. *What to Remember When Waking: The Disciplines of an Everyday Life*. Sounds True Audio, 2010.

Wilson, Shawn. *Research Is Ceremony: Indigenous Research Methods*. Fernwood Publishing, 2008.

Winkler, Gershon. *Magic of the Ordinary: Recovering the Shamanic in Judaism*. North Atlantic Books, 2003.

Wolynn, Mark. *It Didn't Start with You: How Inherited Family Trauma Shapes Who We Are and How to End the Cycle*. Viking, 2016.

Yehuda, Rachel, and Amy Lehrner. "Intergenerational Transmission of Trauma Effects: Putative Role of Epigenetic Mechanisms." *World Psychiatry* 17, no. 3 (Sept. 2018): 243–57. https://doi.org/10.1002/wps.20568.

Yehuda, Rachel, and Linda M. Bierer. "The Relevance of Epigenetics to PTSD: Implications for the DSM-V." *Journal of Traumatic Stress* 22, no. 5 (Oct. 2009): 427–34. https://doi.org/10.1002/jts.20448.

Yehuda, Rachel, Nikolaos P. Daskalakis, Linda M. Bierer, Heather N. Bader, Torsten Klengel, Florian Holsboer, and Elisabeth B. Binder. "Holocaust Exposure Induced Intergenerational Effects on FKBP5 Methylation." *Biological Psychiatry* 80, no. 5 (Sept. 2016): 372–80. https://doi.org/10.1016/j.biopsych.2015.08.005.

To Write to the Author

If you wish to contact the author or would like more information about this book, please write to the author in care of Llewellyn Worldwide Ltd. and we will forward your request. Both the author and publisher appreciate hearing from you and learning of your enjoyment of this book and how it has helped you. Llewellyn Worldwide Ltd. cannot guarantee that every letter written to the author can be answered, but all will be forwarded. Please write to:

Linda Yael Schiller
℅ Llewellyn Worldwide
2143 Wooddale Drive
Woodbury, MN 55125-2989

Please enclose a self-addressed stamped envelope for reply, or $1.00 to cover costs. If outside the U.S.A., enclose an international postal reply coupon.

Many of Llewellyn's authors have websites with additional information and resources. For more information, please visit our website at http://www.llewellyn.com.